Sober Love

Sober Love

How to Quit Drinking as a Couple

Joseph Nowinski, PhD

Foreword by Marvin D. Seppala, MD
Former Chief Medical Officer, Hazelden Betty Ford Foundation

JOHNS HOPKINS UNIVERSITY PRESS | *Baltimore*

Note to the reader: The names and personal details of the individuals and couples featured in this book have been altered to preserve their privacy and confidentiality. Similarly, conversations included in the book have been paraphrased and not quoted verbatim.

Johns Hopkins University Press
2715 North Charles Street
Baltimore, Maryland 21218
www.press.jhu.edu

Library of Congress Cataloging-in-Publication Data

Names: Nowinski, Joseph, author. | Seppala, Marvin D., foreword author.
Title: Sober love : how to quit drinking as a couple / by Joseph Nowinski, PhD;
    foreword by Marvin D. Seppala, MD.
Description: Baltimore : Johns Hopkins University Press, [2024] | Series:
    A Johns Hopkins press health book | Includes bibliographical references
    and index.
Identifiers: LCCN 2023049886 | ISBN 9781421449142 (hardcover) |
    ISBN 9781421449159 (paperback) | ISBN 9781421449166 (ebook)
Subjects: LCSH: Alcoholism. | Temperance. | Couples—Alcohol use.
Classification: LCC HV5060 .N69 2024 | DDC 362.292—
    dc23/eng/20231106
LC record available at https://lccn.loc.gov/2023049886

A catalog record for this book is available from the British Library.

Special discounts are available for bulk purchases of this book.
For more information, please contact Special Sales at specialsales@jh.edu.

For my family:
Theresa
Maggie, Rebecca, and Gregory
With Love and Gratitude

CONTENTS

FOREWORD

IT'S A GREAT PLEASURE to introduce this remarkable book by Joseph Nowinski, PhD. As an addiction psychiatrist who has worked in substance use disorder treatment throughout my career, I have provided care to individuals and families with both substance use disorders and mental health problems. After more than 20 years as chief medical officer of the Hazelden Betty Ford Foundation, where I was responsible for all clinical programs and services, I retired in December 2021. These days, I see people with substance use disorders in a private practice, do some consulting, and provide medical expert work. I also regularly receive calls from people asking about substance use disorders among family members, often a spouse.

I have known and respected Dr. Nowinski for decades. He wrote *The Twelve Step Facilitation Therapy Manual* for Project MATCH, defining Twelve-Step facilitation therapy for research purposes, and later wrote a handbook on the same subject for Hazelden Publications. The research from Project MATCH proved the significant benefits of this therapy, and his books established a standard for the addiction field by formalizing a therapy that utilized the Twelve Steps of Alcoholics Anonymous. Our paths crossed at the Hazelden Betty Ford Foundation, and our careers in addiction treatment overlap considerably in that we both provided clinical care, supervised other clinicians, taught about addiction and its treatment, and administrated addiction programs.

Alcohol use disorders are complex, stigmatized problems. Few people understand these issues, poor advice abounds, and expertise is hard to find. Most physicians receive no more than eight hours of training on these disorders during medical school. Most psychologists have similar limitations; social workers and nurses have even less experience treating alcohol use disorders. Our mental health and medical systems are often ill prepared to care for people who have a problem with alcohol. Neglected in the alcohol use disorders literature are couples, whose relationships may be threatened by drinking. For anyone who wants to change their relationship with drinking—and their partner—but doesn't know where to turn, *Sober Love* may be just the resource they need to start making that change.

In this book, Dr. Nowinski, a highly qualified expert who uses the latest research and his clinical experience to care for people with alcohol issues, provides essential information for couples seeking help. Written for those couples who recognize alcohol has interfered with their lives and want solutions, *Sober Love* focuses on both a couple's commitment to each other and to sober love, or abstinence from alcohol. This recommendation of abstinence is based upon clinical research, the author's years of experience working with couples, and the increasing scientific evidence any amount of alcohol can be harmful to health. Commitment to sobriety may seem like a difficult decision, but it is essential to recommitting to and healing many relationships. Dr. Nowinski provides the information necessary to develop and carry out a plan for both members of the relationship to stop drinking and to establish sober love.

Sober Love provides readers with sage, easily understood advice directly from an expert. Dr. Nowinski offers clear, practical, workable solutions for those couples finding themselves adversely altered by regular alcohol use. He does not provide a magical, singular solution for all couples, because it does not exist. Instead, he provides questions for couples to ask themselves, guiding them to examine and discuss their particular situation, and then offers potential paths forward. Throughout the book are multiple examples from his experience working with diverse couples dealing with problems linked to alcohol.

Without attention, problematic alcohol use can undermine even the best of relationships. This book delivers the information necessary to develop a plan to discontinue alcohol and heal your relationship. Dr. Nowinski guides you with expert knowledge, experience, and care to solutions that work. I will be providing this book to my patients.

Marvin D. Seppala, MD
Former Chief Medical Officer
Hazelden Betty Ford Foundation

Sober Love

Introduction

WHY THIS BOOK, AND WHY NOW?

IN AMERICA TODAY, we face an epidemic of harm from opioids. According to the National Institute for Health Statistics, more than a million people in the United States have died from drug overdoses since 1999. In 2021 alone, there were more than 100,000 overdose deaths attributed to opioids. These statistics have given rise to "harm reduction" efforts, including the widespread availability of Narcan, an opioid antagonist that can be administered by anyone and that can reverse the effects of an opioid overdose. Such emergency interventions can and do save lives. But there has not been a commensurate effort to fund and enhance longer-term treatment programs to help the victims of opioid dependence get a toe hold on a substance-free lifestyle.

As bad as the numbers on opioid-related deaths are, the data relative to drinking are worse. In fact, alcohol accounts for even more deaths than opioids—more than 140,000 a year, according to the Centers for Disease Control and Prevention. Perhaps worse, the National Institute on Alcohol Abuse and Alcoholism reports that "approximately 389,000 of hospital discharges annually for persons 12 and older had a principal alcohol-related diagnosis."

The truth is, Americans drink a lot. They drink so much that *The Atlantic* magazine was moved to run a lead story with the ominous title, "America Has a Drinking Problem." Bolstered by government statistics like those above, the writer reached the following conclusion: "A little alcohol can boost creativity and strengthen social ties. But there's nothing moderate, or convivial, about the way many Americans drink today."

A recent major study looked into the truth behind the common belief that so-called moderate drinking, generally understood as having one or two drinks a day, can be beneficial to a person's health. But what constitutes a drink? The National Institute on Alcohol Abuse and Alcoholism defines a "standard drink" as one that contains 14 grams of alcohol. Using this measure, the researchers of this massive study, which looked at nearly 5 million participants, "found no significant reductions in risk of all-cause mortality for drinkers who drank less than 25 g of ethanol per day" (about 2 standard drinks). "Meaning: Low-volume alcohol drinking was not associated with protection against death from all causes."

So much for this popular myth.

It's not an exaggeration to say that America today is awash in alcohol. As drinking increasingly poses challenges to health and circumstances, the time may come when a couple is ready to take stock of the role that drinking plays in their lives—including the effect on their relationship—and consider changing direction. In other words, this is a book for couples who are ready to be honest about how drinking is affecting their relationship, with an eye toward considering becoming a sober couple.

That some couples share a drinking problem is beyond doubt. Though many people say they know this intuitively, researchers in the field of substance misuse treatment have only recently begun to shed light on the unique effects alcohol has on relationships. Truth be told, they mostly came upon this evidence accidentally, while not really looking for it. These researchers wanted to see if women seeking treatment for a drinking problem (or "alcohol use disorder") would have better outcomes if their husbands or live-in partners were included in treatment, as compared to women who were treated by themselves. So, they recruited women who met this criterion and assessed their partners' drinking habits as well. To their surprise, in one study, 38% of those women who were recruited for treatment had to be excluded because their partners also had a drinking problem. In another study, 70% of couples had to be eliminated for the same reason. These staggering numbers are evidence of a problem on a wide scale—one that has received scant attention until now.

In 2000, one pair of researchers designed an intervention called Behavioral Couples Therapy, or BCT, to treat "co-occurring" drinking problems. In their intervention, spouses who did not have a drinking problem were enlisted to provide support and reinforcement (encouragement, praise) for the drinking partner who was trying to quit. They reported some success with this approach, but they hastened to add that BCT was not effective when both spouses had a drinking problem. Their intervention was aimed at helping only one partner, not both. Little wonder it was only effective that way.

A joint decision to become a sober couple amounts to a major change in direction (and identity) for a couple. They may make this decision after realizing that drinking has progressively deprived their relationships of vitality, intimacy, and direction. In effect, drinking *hollows out* a relationship in ways that will be described in this book. The good news, though, is that there is a solution to a shared drinking problem. *Sober Love* offers couples ways to reverse that hollowing and improve their relationship.

There may not be a better time for this book. The past several decades have witnessed a virtual explosion in effective treatments for substance use disorders, including drinking. I have been personally involved in some of that research, including developing an evidence-based treatment model for helping individuals reverse a drinking problem. This approach, along with others that have been developed, can be meaningfully used by couples who acknowledge the role that drinking has come to play in their relationship and are ready to try an alternative lifestyle. Given the pervasive and destructive role that drinking plays in our contemporary culture, there may be no time like the present to pursue this option.

HOW TO USE THIS BOOK

This book is aimed at couples who decide to pursue sobriety together. Its chapters identify and address a range of issues that couples pursuing a sober relationship may encounter, along with specific guidelines for dealing with them as a team. The appendix includes notes and references to the material cited in the text, along with additional resources. This information will be useful to readers who would like to learn about the research, issues, and strategies described here in more detail.

The evidence-based treatment strategies in this book have proven to be effective for people wanting to achieve sobriety. Throughout are case studies of couples I have had the privilege of working with toward achieving this goal. They share their past experiences with drinking, what they needed to do to achieve their goal of sobriety, and the difference it made in their lives moving forward. As the stories told here show, every couple's path to a sober relationship is unique, and something they should be proud to have negotiated together.

I also provide information that sheds light on why America's "drinking problem" has complex causes and is not merely the result of genetics. Readers will learn about the *drinking spectrum* and have the opportunity to assess where they fall on it. Even if the two people in a relationship find themselves at different points along the spectrum, the information in this book can help improve their relationship, which can be thought of as a "third party" that lives alongside them as individuals.

The times we live in may be ripe for a decision to pursue sober love. If you and your partner are thinking of giving sobriety a try, may this book be the starting point you need.

Chapter 1

IT'S ABOUT LOVE

THIS IS A BOOK ABOUT LOVE. It is a book for couples who care enough—not only about themselves, but also about their partner and their relationship—to pursue a sober relationship. This book will be their guide to getting there, and the journey will be worth it.

This is also a book about drinking. That's not to say that either partner in a relationship choosing to move toward sober love drinks to the extent that they would qualify for a traditional diagnosis of alcoholism. At the same time, it is probably true that neither of them drinks at what could be called a low-risk or minimal level. Often, they fall at different points on what is known as the drinking spectrum (figure 1.1).

The decision to pursue a sober relationship depends primarily on several things: how much and how often each partner drinks, how their drinking has affected them both individually and as a couple, and how motivated they are to change their lifestyle in the interest of a better relationship. None of these factors alone may be enough to base a decision on, but taken together, they may point in one direction or another: the status quo, or change. To begin this process of decision-making, let's get an idea of where each partner in a relationship falls with respect to how much they drink.

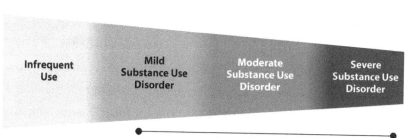

| Infrequent Use | Mild Substance Use Disorder | Moderate Substance Use Disorder | Severe Substance Use Disorder |

Substance Use Disorder

FIGURE 1.1

The drinking spectrum depicts how alcohol use disorder progresses over time. The stages of alcohol use blend into one another, reflecting the way misuse advances, as opposed to being sharply defined categories.

I devised the above diagram of the drinking spectrum to depict how the use of alcohol (and other substances) typically progresses over time in men and women. It has become a standard in the field and is used by clinicians to help clients decide on a diagnosis and a course of action. Couples can use the diagram to determine where they each fall on the spectrum and what they might consider doing next.

Notice, first, that the different areas on the spectrum are not separated by sharp lines; rather, they tend to blend into one another. That is the way that most substance misuse progresses—gradually, and slowly, over time. That tends to be the way it is for drinking. One or two cocktails, glasses of wine, or a few hard ciders or beers on the weekend gradually progresses to multiple drinks every night. And so on. In the diagram, "infrequent use" is equivalent to what professionals and agencies like the National Institute on Alcohol Abuse and Alcoholism (NIAAA) call "low-risk" drinking, meaning a level of drinking associated with few if any significant negative consequences.

The progression of alcohol use can be so slow and insidious that the drinker barely notices it. At its lowest level (infrequent use), there may be no noticeable negative consequences. Infrequent use or drinking only a small amount may have the effect of helping a person unwind from a hard day at work or to ease social situations. Individuals whose drinking ranks them in the infrequent zone typically do not drink daily (or even weekly), and they rarely drink alone. They do not worry about having liquor available, and they are comfortable in social situations where there is little to no drinking. Consequently, they may socialize with a number of sober friends and couples, and they are likely to take care that the partner who drives home from a social engagement is sober.

This is a book about relationships, and it's therefore fitting to translate the drinking spectrum in terms of a relationship. In that respect, drinking at the low-risk or infrequent level on the spectrum can be thought of as a "casual friendship" with alcohol. Casual friendships tend not to take up too much space in a person's (or in this case a couple's) overall lifestyle. They do not compete with other relationships or commitments. In other words, low-risk drinking does not encroach on other areas of life, such as intimacy, family, favored activities, or work.

Now, notice that the spectrum tapers as it moves from left to right. This reflects another reality: most people who drink beyond the low-risk level constitute what are known as "problem drinkers," as compared to the fewer numbers who would qualify as alcoholics (*severe* substance use disorder). As drinking progresses, consequences begin to appear, although most people will not initially "connect the dots" between their gradual increase in drinking and its negative effects, such as being charged with driving under the influence (DUI) or perhaps sustaining an accidental injury.

As individuals and couples move to the right on the spectrum, the nature of their drinking habits also progresses to the mild and moderate zones, where it could rightly be called a *relationship*. The further to the right they are on in the spectrum, the stronger that relationship is. As opposed to a casual friendship, any true relationship a person has occupies a significant space in their lifestyle. As such, the relationship with alcohol competes with other relationships, eventually displacing them more and more. That is exactly what happens as drinking progresses along the spectrum. It affects us as individuals, then distorts our lifestyle and affects our other relationships.

If you take a few minutes to reflect on how your drinking—both as individuals and as a couple—has changed over time, you may be able to see it has moved from being a casual friendship to a relationship. If that is true, how has it affected your other relationships, including your primary relationship with one another? Has one or both of you felt jealous at times about drinking and the space it takes up in your partner's life? Can you look back and recognize that drinking has taken up progressively more space in your life, displacing intimacy, shared pleasures, and even social activities?

At the extreme end of the spectrum (meaning a severe drinking problem, or alcoholism), a person needs to drink in order to feel "normal." At this point, one could say that they are truly "committed" to drinking. They need to have some amount of alcohol circulating in their body; otherwise, they feel out of sorts. They worry about running out of liquor and will often stock up and even stash liquor around the house, in the glove compartment of their car, or in their desk at work. They sleep poorly and are chronically fatigued, and over time they lose any real interests beyond drinking. They will avoid social occasions and places where alcohol is not available, and other relationships take a back seat to drinking, which leads to resentment and eventually to alienation. It is at this point that significant medical problems may arise.

Even for people at the severe end of the spectrum, there are strategies that can help, including the use of medications to diminish cravings. If one partner in a relationship is drinking at that level and the other falls somewhere in the moderate zone, their path to sober love as a couple needs to take that difference into account.

Focusing again on the middle zones of the drinking spectrum, it's critical to understand that individuals and couples do not simply jump from one zone to another; rather, the progression is slow and insidious. It most often begins at the low-risk end, when drinking becomes part of a couple's routine. It may only be one or two drinks, and not every day. That said, some people report, that starting from their very first drink, they could not stop until they got drunk. But that's the exception to the rule. Others still say that they were already somewhere in the mild to moderate zone at the outset of their relationship, and that their partner gradually joined them there. Buying beer, wine, or spirits becomes a routine part of shopping for individuals and couples who enjoy a relationship with drinking. Neither partner may worry much about just how much is in their supply. Gradually, however, over time, the couple begins to look forward to having a drink or two on a regular basis, and usually at a designated time and place. They take pains to make sure they have their favorite liquors available.

What are some of the consequences associated with drinking at the mild to moderate levels? Here are a few of the more common ones, and they will vary in severity depending on just how far a person or couple has drifted along the spectrum:

- Disrupted sleep. Drinking may initially help a person get to sleep, but as the alcohol wears off, they will often wake up early and have difficulty getting back to sleep.

- Feeling sluggish as opposed to refreshed after a night of poor sleep
- Weight gain
- More frequent bowel problems (diarrhea)
- Increased blood pressure or a diagnosis of prediabetes
- Periodic forgetfulness
- Skin problems (poor complexion)
- Feeling easily fatigued
- Gradual loss of interest in once pleasurable activities
- Lethargy (a tendency to sit around as opposed to getting things done)

Take a look at the above list. Experiencing any of these symptoms could indicate a mild drinking problem. And make no mistake—even a mild drinking problem is potentially harmful, both for your health and for your relationship, even if a couple chooses to avoid thinking much about it.

As drinking progresses along the spectrum, its consequences gradually become more apparent, although for many men and women it isn't until they are well into the moderate zone or at the edge of the severe end of the spectrum that the connection between drinking and how it has affected them and their relationship becomes more obvious and difficult to deny. Some severe consequences include:

- Problems at work: declining performance evaluations, absenteeism
- Medical problems: hypertension, renal problems, elevated liver panels
- Legal problems: DUI
- Emotional effects: irritability, depression
- Neglecting usual responsibilities around the home

- Declining intimacy, including affection and sex
- Injuries related to drinking
- Having a friend, family member, or coworker comment on your drinking
- Feeling uncomfortable at times about your own drinking

As a couple, reflect on these consequences of severe drinking and ask yourselves whether any apply to you, your partner, or both. We are not looking for a definitive clinical diagnosis here, but instead a sense of where you are in terms of the drinking spectrum. Should either of you have an interest in doing a more detailed assessment, you can find references to materials for doing so in the appendix.

A HOLLOW TREE

Over time, drinking tends to "hollow out" a relationship and a family as it progresses, just as a parasite can hollow out the core of a tree, gradually weakening it. That said, because drinking does progress slowly along the spectrum, couples may not notice its effects on their relationship or family life for quite some time. Viewed from the outside (by friends, for example), the hollowing out may not be obvious, and the relationship (or family) may appear to be just fine. But once one or both partners progress to the moderate level, they should be able to look back, take stock, and see how drinking has affected their lives.

Here are some ways a moderate problem drinking affects a relationship over time:

- Less time spent simply communicating: sharing the day's activities, talking about current events, planning for the future
- Loss of intimacy: hugging, cuddling, sex

- More time leading "parallel lives": doing things separately (including at home) as opposed to together
- Loss of interest in previously rewarding activities: watching movies, playing games, gardening
- Fatigue: heading to bed early
- Chronic irritability, frustration, and impatience
- More frequent spats

If a couple has children, add these to the list of consequences associated with moderate drinking problems in one or both partners:

- Less time interacting with children: reading, talking, doing things together
- Less time monitoring schoolwork
- Less enforcement of limits and house rules
- More frequent parent-child conflict
- Fewer family activities
- Children spending more time either isolated in the house or out of the house
- Children rarely if ever inviting friends over

As we move into that part of the book that explores the effects of drinking on relationships and family life more deeply, readers will find examples that illustrate this hollowing-out process. For now, reflect on the above lists. Which if any of these effects can you identify with?

An exact diagnosis is less important than recognizing that you both fall somewhere along the spectrum—maybe not in the severe range, but not in the infrequent range, either. Based on that self-assessment, you can consider whether you as a couple are open to the idea of a sober relationship.

Taken together, the effects of drinking on the individual, the relationship, and the family are good grist for the mill when thinking about whether to pursue sober love, and whether choosing to become a sober couple offers an opportunity for a more satisfying lifestyle for all concerned. In other words, the decision to contemplate is this: Would our relationship (and perhaps our family) be enhanced if we decided to become a sober couple?

Chapter 2

WHY WE DRINK

WE AMERICANS DRINK A LOT. In this chapter, we examine why and how so many people (and by extension couples) are vulnerable to slipping into a pattern of drinking too much, moving progressively from the low-risk into the mild and moderate zones of the drinking spectrum. At the same time, we need to take a more critical look at one of the reasons why it can be so difficult for individuals and couples to face up to their drinking: the stigma that is still associated with the idea of having a "drinking problem."

One common belief about drinking that plays into this stigma is that drinking and alcoholism are caused by our genes, meaning that if we drink too much, we can blame heredity. But that view is too narrow. The truth is that while our genes may play a role, they are far from the determining factor in how we progress along the drinking spectrum. Drinking problems have multifaceted causes, and couples who understand this will have an easier time getting past any stigma that may stand in their way. Being aware of the various factors involved in alcohol use disorder can also help couples anticipate potential pitfalls as they move toward sober love.

Why we drink turns out to be complicated. Let's look at some of the influences—aside from genetics—on our drinking.

THE DRINKING CULTURE

Most Western cultures are soaked in drinking culture. In the United States, the liquor industry is predicted to spend a whopping $7.7 billion in advertising in 2023, which is up from the $6.7 billion it spent in 2020. Alcohol brands spend twice as much on television as the average brand and nearly four times as much on "out-of-home" advertising (social media, magazines, billboards, etc.). So-called digital advertising (which appears on the Internet and streaming television) is set to account for 30% of alcohol advertising spending in 2023.

This level of saturation affects not only adults, but youths as well. For example, a three-year study of magazine advertising found that 23.1% of ads for adult alcoholic beverages appeared in magazines with high youth readership, and almost double that number (42.9%) of ads aimed at youths were placed in the same magazines. Young people in markets where there is a saturation of alcohol advertising tend to increase their alcohol consumption over time to the point where many consume an average of 50 drinks per month by age 25.

The bottom line of all this advertising boils down to this: the more advertising young people see, the more they drink. No wonder, then, that one reason we drink is our culture that promotes it, much like it once promoted smoking, which most people at the time also started early in life, believing it was harmless.

Why does this matter? As a couple reading this book, and contemplating moving forward to shared sobriety, you can expect the drinking culture to exert its effects on you—in particular, on urges you may experience to have a drink. Some of these urges may be physical in nature (a gut craving), but they are equally likely to take the form of an unconscious thought in response to an image you see. Television, the Internet, and other social media are saturated with ads that make drinking not just appealing, but also desirable. They equate drinking with having fun and being social. They play on a natural desire to be a "normal" adult, to fit in with the socially acceptable drinking culture.

The data on liquor advertising aimed at youths are worrisome. Liquor companies make efforts to appeal to young people by marketing types of liquor—flavored hard seltzer, for example, and hard cider—that they believe will make drinking more appealing. This seems to work, as half of all drinkers who went on to develop alcohol dependence report that their drinking careers started at age 16 or younger.

If you decide that it's in your best interest to work toward, say, a year of being a sober couple, you can expect our drinking culture to exploit any urges you may experience to have that martini (or beer, or wine) you don't want to miss out on. Media such as television and print advertising may also reinforce the idea that being sober is "abnormal." To prepare for the challenges of our drinking culture, ask yourselves the following questions and then share your thoughts with your partner:

- Considering all the advertising messages you get, from television to print and online media, are you inclined on some level to believe that drinking is part of being a "normal" person and that not drinking is somehow "abnormal"?
- Have your liquor preferences been influenced by advertising that promotes one brand over another, or one type over another?
- Have you been vulnerable to ads that suggest some forms of alcohol (such as hard cider or flavored hard seltzer) are essentially harmless, even healthy?
- When you see an ad for liquor, do you find yourself wanting a drink?

This idea of drinking as normal and sobriety as abnormal is central to the drinking culture, but it is not universal. Some cultures (such as Muslim ones and New Order Amish in the United States) regard abstinence as normal and desirable. The temperance movement that once was popular in Europe and the United States also advocated abstinence and associated drinking with various social evils, including rising spousal and child abuse rates. Today, some subcultures ritualize drinking; in other words, drinking is considered normal on certain occasions, but drinking on a regular basis is not.

The above can be good food for thought as you and your partner reflect on your relationship with alcohol and each other, how you may have been influenced by the drinking culture, and what if any changes you are contemplating together. For example, you could make a game out of identifying ads for drinking, pointing them out to one another, and laughing at how they try to normalize drinking even as they say, "Please drink responsibly!"

THE PSYCHOLOGY OF DRINKING

Just as there is a cultural aspect behind drinking, there is a psychological component as well. Most people are motivated to begin their drinking careers for one or both of the following reasons:

- To promote a positive emotional state
- To mute a negative emotional state

Carolyn Knapp, in her bestselling memoir *Drinking: A Love Story*, succinctly captures both psychological motives for drinking this way: "I loved the way drink could shift my attention onto something less painful than my own feelings and the warming, melting feelings of ease and courage it gave me." On the one hand, Knapp drank to quell whatever emotional demons had haunted her, apparently for a long time. On the other hand, drinking led to feelings of comfort and helped her to be more assertive and outgoing.

People have turned to drinking to deal with their emotions for generations. History (like Knapp's autobiography) tells us, however, that using alcohol to cope with life's ups and downs does not work in the long run. Many people who find themselves drinking excessively often identify more with one psychological motive than the other. For example, adult survivors of emotional or sexual abuse as children may say that drinking helps to mute the feelings of anxiety and shame that are the result of those experiences. But there are other psychological factors as well.

HARRY AND JILL

Harry had a severe stutter as a child, which resulted in heavy teasing and ridicule from his peers. Though the stutter had been treated and was no more than a mild issue by the time Harry started college, he nevertheless developed a habit of drinking before and during social events, as he found that it facilitated his ability to interact with others. He typically continued drinking and often got drunk on such occasions, though he believed he had a high tolerance for alcohol and that others could not tell.

In his first year after graduating, Harry started up a relationship with Jill, a teacher with whom he felt more comfortable than he'd ever been with a romantic interest. But she too had a habit of drinking before and during social events, as a way of compensating for some mild but long-standing social anxiety. Unlike Harry, though, Jill rarely drank to the point of becoming drunk.

After dating for six months, Jill shared her concern with Harry about his habit of drinking before social events or avoiding them if he couldn't drink ahead of time. She also confided that she noticed he would continue to drink a lot once they got there. Though Harry didn't think she could tell, Jill knew when he was drunk. She acknowledged her own reliance on alcohol as a social facilitator, to compensate for some social shyness, and she admitted she was not fond of this dependence. This led to a conversation about the role that drinking had come to play in both their lives. Then Jill told Harry that she valued their relationship and had thought about a possible future together, but she was worried about his (and her) drinking. Her own mother, she said, had a severe drinking problem that had rendered her unavailable and ineffective as a parent, and Jill was aware and wary of the destructive role that drinking could play in a relationship and family. With that in mind, Jill said she wanted to take a break from their relationship.

Jill and Harry's story shows that some of the motives to drink typically have roots in a person's early life but tend to persist into adulthood. In their cases, neither was yet at a point that could be described as alcoholism, but neither were they at the low-risk part of the spectrum.

In reflecting on the above, ask yourself the following questions, which may offer insight as to why you drink:

- Have you ever felt shame about something in your life? What events or circumstances caused you to have those feelings? Do you believe that drinking may have helped you to "mute" that shame?
- Have you ever used alcohol to compensate for any anxiety— social or otherwise—that you experience? Do you sometimes use alcohol as a social facilitator?

GENES AND DRINKING

Research on the genetics of drinking has focused on individuals whose drinking falls on the severe end of the drinking spectrum, or what is commonly called alcoholism. These people have reached a point in their drinking where they must have some alcohol in their bodies to feel normal. Without it, they experience a great deal of discomfort along with a craving to drink. They tend to store up alcohol so as not to run out, and they may even resort to keeping some in the glove compartment or their handbag. They also are likely to have experienced serious consequences due to drinking: to their health, their work, their relationships.

For this group of drinkers at least, researchers have established a clear connection within families. Surveys have consistently found, for example, that first-degree relatives (parents, siblings, or children) of those who have been treated for alcoholism are two to four times more likely to be alcoholics than the relatives of nonalcoholics. Meanwhile, studies of identical twins have shown that if one twin is an alcoholic, the other twin has a roughly 50% chance of also being an alcoholic.

As much as these data should be a wake-up call for readers from families with a history of substance use disorders, it is not inevitable that everyone will develop such problems. Even among identical twins, for example, where the genetic risk appears to be greatest, there is a 50% chance that the twin of an alcoholic will *not* become an alcoholic. The difference may be that these individuals heed the warning signs and either refrain from substance use or take pains to stay in the low-risk zone. It also will depend on the kind of lifestyle they may have developed and whether it also tends to support sobriety or at least low-risk use.

What lesson should we take from this information? Both partners in a relationship would be wise to realize that they may be at increased risk for sliding further into the drinking spectrum if alcoholism runs in their families. At the same time, it is far from inevitable. Making a decision to become a sober couple is a sure way to avoid even the possibility that this could happen to one or both partners.

SOCIAL NETWORKS AND DRINKING

Virtually everyone these days uses social media. Platforms like Facebook, X, Instagram, TikTok, and others exert a strong influence on the information we receive, which in turn can influence our beliefs and our behavior. In fact, the combined influence of social networks probably outweighs the influence of advertising. As these platforms present drinking—and other substance use—as benign, the idea of a sober lifestyle may seem boring in comparison to a drinking lifestyle.

For most of us, the most powerful social network that influences our behavior is the one that is most immediate: family, friends, and sometimes coworkers. Many people who find themselves further along on the drinking spectrum state that they previously had a fairly diverse social network. In other words, they had friends and associates who were nondrinkers as well as low-risk drinkers. Over time, however, these moderate drinkers' social networks gradually changed, eventually matching their own alcohol use. As the people and situations around them changed, heavy drinking slowly became reinforced and normalized.

For some people, immediate family constitutes a mini-drinking culture in itself. If this situation applies to you, presenting your relationship as a sober couple can be challenging. It can make other family members uncomfortable, and even lead to you or your partner being teased or pressured to "have just one."

Most couples who choose to pursue sober love will need to make at least some modifications to their social network. It may be time to forego the ritual Friday after-work happy hour. Meeting friends (at least, drinking friends) at the local sports bar may need to stop. But deciding to pursue a sober relationship may also involve reconnecting with sober friends who've dropped out of your social network. For others, fellowships like Alcoholics Anonymous (AA), Secular AA, Women for Sobriety, and Self-Management and Recovery Training (SMART) Recovery offer avenues where couples can receive respect and support for choosing sober love.

BOTTOM LINE: IT'S COMPLICATED

The purpose for including this discussion is simple: it debunks any simplistic explanation for why people drink. Gradually sliding along the drinking spectrum from low-risk, to mild, to moderate, to severe drinking is not solely the result of genetics, past trauma, or social networks. But all of these areas of our lives are associated with the consequences of alcohol use, even the mild ones toward the left of the spectrum. In fact, the initial consequences of a developing drinking problem may be so subtle and gradual that drinkers don't recognize them. Eventually, though—as we will see in the next chapter—it becomes more difficult to deny those connections.

For now, couples might reflect on and talk to one another about the above factors and how they may play a role in each partner's drinking. It may also help to discuss roughly where on the drinking spectrum each partner believes they are today.

Chapter 3

COUPLES WHO CHOSE SOBER LOVE

BEFORE MOVING ON, let's take some time to look at some of the couples who have chosen sober love over the drinking life. As you'll see, they are diverse both in terms of where each partner fell on the drinking spectrum and in terms of their lifestyles and the issues they faced.

SUSAN AND JAKE

"I honestly don't know which one of us was more miserable in the end," said Susan. "Jake had just gotten his first DUI, despite the fact that he'd been driving intoxicated for years and gotten away with it. And I had just finished mandatory DUI classes after getting my own DUI, even though I was barely over the legal limit when I got stopped by police. To top it off, my doctor warned me that my latest annual revealed that my liver was showing some early warning signs and questioned me about my drinking. My father had died from sclerosis, and that really scared me."

Married for 18 years, Jake and Susan had a 16-year-old son and a 13-year-old daughter. Their son, Matt, had been diagnosed with attention deficit disorder at age 8 and had been on medication since. The medication helped, and the disruptive behavior and learning problems that had marked his first years in school had improved, but he was still prone to distraction, had trouble remembering things his parents asked him to do, and was generally academically unmotivated.

Matt's sister, Madelyn, in contrast, was an academic star and an athlete. But after her latest physical, the pediatrician sat both Maddie and Susan down and told them that Maddie was significantly underweight for her age and height and that she wanted to see her again in six months. For Susan, the comment raised the ominous specter of anorexia. She had a friend whose daughter had an eating disorder, and it had been a nightmare. Susan dreaded the possibility that her own daughter might fall into that trap as well.

The challenges that Jake and Susan faced at this stage in their lives and marriage—children, careers, and maintaining a home—are not all that unusual. But in their case, a shared involvement with alcohol was very much a complicating factor. Not all couples dealing with such challenges feel overwhelmed, but Susan did, and drinking played a role. Over time, she felt she had less and less energy. She also had put on weight, and her complexion had become what she described as rather pale and lifeless. Her interest in sex had declined over the past few years, and though Jake rarely complained, the fact was that sex between them had gradually dwindled to the point of being almost nonexistent. The same was true for time spent sitting together: watching a show on television, cuddling on the family room couch, or just talking were things they rarely did together anymore.

For his part, Jake felt frustrated by his son's lack of motivation and less-than-average academic performance—especially since both Jake and Susan had earned degrees and were engaged in successful careers, he as a financial adviser and she as a marketing executive.

One night, after both kids had retreated to their respective bedrooms and Susan had consumed her usual three glasses of wine, she asked Jake if he thought they each had a drinking problem. She'd been contemplating the possibility off and on since her physical exam and the liver report. But then Jake's DUI brought it to a head for her, and while he seemed to want to avoid talking, Susan insisted. It was the first time they, as a couple, broke through what you might call "the shared secret" of a drinking problem.

Both Susan and Jake started their drinking careers fairly early in life. Alcoholism ran a clear pathway through Jake's family tree. His father was a heavy drinker and suffered from several medical complications, including hypertension and diabetes. Though he no longer drank, Jake's father had paid for his drinking career, as he now faced physical limitations. Jake had started drinking at around age 14 and never really stopped. Like Susan, his drinking accelerated during his college years, tapered off somewhat after he got his first job, but then gradually increased again over the ensuing years.

Susan's drinking really began only after she and Jake started attending the same university. They saw each other on a number of occasions—usually at parties where heavy drinking occurred—but didn't date until a year later. By then, Susan was well into the weekend partying scene at the school. On one occasion she had gotten drunk, passed out, and the next morning woke up in bed next to a male student she didn't know. That scared her, but not enough to move her to quit. Later, she faced a similar incident when she found herself in the back seat of a car with two male students who were in the act of removing her clothes. On that occasion she was alert enough to scream and resist, so the boys let her out of the car half naked.

Soon after that incident, Susan began dating Jake. While she never again experienced another compromising situation, she did not stop drinking (though she did drink less). That pattern initially defined their adult relationship, though it included regularly consuming beer, wine, occasional cocktails, and more recently hard seltzer or cider. Susan had to admit, at least to herself, that over time both she and Jake regularly drank to a point that she described as just short of intoxication, two or three nights a week, and on other nights they rarely abstained entirely.

Susan was the one who took the initiative to seek counseling about her drinking, but Jake said he wasn't really interested. He did own up to his DUI but insisted that it was a "random event" and not a sign of a real problem.

Through counseling, Susan was able to do an honest assessment of herself in relation to drinking and concluded that alcohol had become like a "relationship" alongside her relationship with Jake in her life. She'd never intended for that to happen, but she could see how it had crept up on her over time. Moreover, it had led to consequences that previously she had not attributed to their true cause: drinking. These included not just the unsettling liver issue, but also a slow decline in energy and general vitality, a gradually disappearing sex life, and less time spent simply interacting with Jake. Whereas early in their relationship she and Jake took great pleasure in working on jigsaw puzzles together, as well as playing chess and board games—Scrabble being a favorite—those games were now gathering dust in the closet. Susan and Jake also had enjoyed hiking and cross-country skiing with their kids. But over the past two years they'd gone skiing only once as a family. Similarly, Susan's counselor made her aware of two additional changes: the fact that she now rarely asked Madelyn or Matt how they were doing in school, despite Matt's clear issue of underachievement, plus the fact that both kids avoided inviting friends over to the house.

When Susan first announced to Jake that she'd reached a decision to quit drinking for 90 days, he asked her if she thought she had a problem. She said yes, then asked him if he thought the same was true for him. He said no, adding that if she wanted to quit that was fine, but that he still believed that any consequences that correlated with his drinking were mere coincidences. If Susan had a "drinking problem," so be it, but Jake could hold his liquor. Jake's thinking about drinking would eventually change, however.

A few months later, Jake headed out to retrieve Madelyn from her middle school volleyball game. It was about six o'clock in the evening, and as usual he'd already consumed three cans of spiked cider (after a flavored martini). While backing out from their driveway, he failed to see an oncoming vehicle, which hit the rear of his car. That left Susan to fetch her daughter while the driver of the other car insisted on reporting the accident to police. Needless to say, Jake sweated the whole time they waited for the trooper to arrive. Lucky for him, the trooper simply wrote out a report and didn't ask Jake to take a sobriety test. Had he failed one, Jake was facing likely jail time for a second DUI.

After the accident—in another conversation initiated by Susan—Jake told Susan that he would "cut down" on his drinking, specifically that he would forego martinis and wine in favor of "just some hard seltzer." But within a month he was consuming an entire six-pack or more of hard seltzer every day, even more than his previous consumption. Then something else happened.

When Jake met with his manager for his annual performance review, he was presented with some disturbing information. First, the anonymous annual ratings left by his clients had significantly declined over the previous year. Second, he was now getting virtually no new clients through referrals from existing ones. The bottom line was that the portfolio of investments he was managing had decreased by several millions of dollars. Under the circumstances, Jake's manager informed him that he would receive no bonus that year, with the expectation moving forward that he would rebuild his portfolio.

When Jake reluctantly shared this news with Susan, she felt she had no choice but to respond by citing Jake's drinking and the results of his failed attempt to cut down. This conversation was tense, especially when Susan shared how difficult she found it to not drink while Jake continued to do so. She told him that there were times when she felt like she was holding on to a fragile sobriety "by my fingernails."

The next day, Jake announced that he would stop drinking for one month. Still, even that resolve lasted only seven days, at which point Jake declared that he "deserved" a martini on a Sunday afternoon. One martini turned into two, plus four cans of hard seltzer, after which Jake fell asleep on the family room couch. Susan found this scene intolerable, leaving to visit a friend while Jake stayed home and drank. By then it was also painfully obvious to her that the children were aware of their father's drinking but chose to avoid talking about it.

Many couples reading this book may be able to relate to Jake and Susan's story. Sadly, the themes that define their situation are more common than many people would care to believe. The dilemma faced by this couple is not that uncommon, regardless of how their lives may differ in other ways. Susan aptly described her relationship with Jake as one of "shared misery," realizing for the first time how the quality of their relationship had diminished over time and how they'd unintentionally conspired to avoid facing that reality.

After a few more heart-to-heart talks, a good deal of reflection, and a couple of talks with Susan's counselor, they decided together to become a sober couple. They felt that this was in the interest of themselves as individuals, of their relationship, and of their family. And so they began their journey.

JOHN AND MARTIN

This longtime couple shared how, over a period of years, they had found themselves gradually purchasing and consuming more and more "top shelf" brands of vodka, which they used to make martinis. They did this, John explained with a laugh, in an effort "to keep up with the Joneses." Their social network was professional and fairly upscale, and one of its status symbols was the vodka used to make martinis at social gatherings. When asked if they could taste the difference between a martini made with a $30 bottle of vodka as opposed to one made with a $50 bottle, they both laughed again. "Of course not!" Martin replied.

John and Martin had decided to pursue shared sobriety for one year after having several talks with a counselor about their drinking. Both attorneys (from different firms), they were successful, co-owned a city townhouse in an upscale neighborhood, and enjoyed a large discretionary income that in the past they had used to fund adventurous vacations as well as an active city life. But there was also a darker side to their affluent lifestyle.

It was Martin who first brought up the idea that their drinking had been progressively getting "out of hand" for at least two years, if not longer. Their work involved—for both of them, sometimes separately, at other times together—a fair amount of socializing, which almost invariably included drinking. Drinking after work had gradually extended to their home life and increased over time, from one martini a night to two and sometimes three. They were also aware that one of their colleagues, an older man, had recently been diagnosed with diabetes that he'd confessed was related to drinking, while another couple had broken up a ten-year relationship, reportedly because of one partner's alcoholism. In looking back on the past couple of years, it became apparent that their once vibrant city life had slowly dwindled. They ate out less often, had not attended a concert or a play in a year, and had no vacation plans in mind.

On reflection, another consequence they could connect to drinking was John's increasing difficulty maintaining an erection when they had sex. John's doctor noted during a recent physical that his blood pressure had increased noticeably over the previous year and discussed the option of prescribing medication. The doctor also inquired about John's alcohol intake. He owned up to his drinking, adding that his own father had died of a heart attack at the age of 52.

John spoke with Martin about his physical. He said he was willing to try medication, but he also brought up the issue of their shared drinking patterns, as well as his own developing sexual dysfunction. At that point they had been a couple for six years and had recently talked about marriage. Martin mentioned the unfortunate consequences that had befallen some of their friends. "You know, if we're honest about it, we could end up like that ourselves," he said. John's initial reaction was to get defensive, saying that he did not believe he was an alcoholic. He also worried about how their friends and colleagues might react if they suddenly stopped drinking. "Don't you think they'd think we were weird?" he asked. So Martin dropped the subject for the moment.

A month later, John and Martin were at yet another of their frequent social gatherings, where expensive wine and martinis were flowing freely. John indulged so much that Martin had to insist on driving home, while John passed out in the car. That prompted another talk the next day. Martin said he didn't know if either of them was truly an alcoholic, but he had no doubt that they were on a mutually destructive path. He then added that he didn't want to get into a marriage where alcoholism might become an issue, as it had been in both his own parents' marriage and that of a younger, now divorced sister. This time John listened, then asked Martin what they should do. Martin replied that he thought they should both get sober for a time, even if that meant having to curtail their social lives. At that point they decided to see a therapist that a good friend had recommended.

SUZANNE AND CINDY

The psychological motives behind disordered drinking typically have their roots in early life but tend to persist well into adulthood. This was certainly true for Suzanne, who began drinking at around age 15, about the same time that it first dawned on her that she might be gay. She knew her family did not approve of homosexuality, so she tried to avoid thinking about it. Stealing whiskey from her father's well-stocked family room bar helped her do just that.

Despite drinking regularly at a young age, Suzanne managed to be a successful student and a better-than-average basketball player. Tall and slender, with a good eye for the basket and a nice release, she made the varsity team in high school and went on to play as a walk-on at the college level. All the while, despite having several platonic relationships with men, she only felt sexual attraction to other women.

During her first college years, Suzanne continued, to use her word, to be "plagued" by feelings of sexual attraction to other women, yet the shame she experienced in association with such feelings prevented her from acting on them. Instead, she dwelled on them internally. And while her fellow college students downed their fair share of beer on weekends, Suzanne kept a bottle of whiskey secretly stashed in her room.

Suzanne's first sexual experience turned out to be with an assistant basketball coach, who was a senior when Suzanne was a sophomore. It began with the two of them drinking at a homecoming weekend party off campus and ended with the two of them making love at the coach's apartment. Suzanne was drunk at the time, explaining that she didn't consciously know what she was doing—she simply surrendered to an urge she'd been resisting for so long.

The relationship with the assistant basketball coach continued on and off for the remainder of that academic year. On returning to campus for her junior year, Suzanne dropped off the basketball team and avoided any more sexual encounters until after graduating with a business degree.

At 30, Suzanne was employed as an accountant. She was once again involved sexually, this time with Cindy, a graphic artist who was employed at the same company, and they'd been partners for three years. Her family was still in the dark about Suzanne's sexuality and knew Cindy only as a roommate. At that point, Suzanne was drinking whiskey or wine every night, with Cindy slowly beginning to catch up. The main reason for the heavy drinking, according to Cindy, was that Suzanne was not able to engage in any physical contact at all—be that hugging, kissing, or sex—unless she was intoxicated. That left Cindy feeling frustrated, as she loved Suzanne very much. So they ended up becoming drinking partners, such that over the course of their relationship, Cindy's drinking had gradually increased to the point where sex was not only infrequent but also dependent on alcohol.

It was Cindy's frustration that finally led them to consult a therapist. And though they sought counseling to address the problem of infrequent sex, plus the fact that Suzanne had difficulty reaching orgasm, drinking soon became the focus of their sessions. The therapist explained to Cindy and Suzanne that while alcohol has long been used to disinhibit sexuality, it also can interfere with the sexual response in men and women. As time passes and drinking becomes ingrained in a relationship, intimacy—including sexual intimacy—erodes as a function of lethargy, decreased vitality, and/or sexual dysfunction.

Aside from the sexual issue, it was apparent that there were more problems in their relationship, including Suzanne's lingering shame about her sexuality, as well as a lifestyle that had progressively hollowed out as the couple's drinking increased. For example, for the first couple of years they were together, Suzanne and Cindy enjoyed an active city life and all it had to offer, including museums, concerts, and fine dining, as well as weekend walks in a nearby park. But most of these things—like intimacy—had gradually fallen by the wayside. Now, if they did go out to eat, they walked to one of a few local bistros to avoid the risk of a DUI. They'd been to an art exhibit only once and to a concert not at all in the past year. Walks in the park were no longer a regular activity either. Now their daily after-work routine began with scotch on the rocks for Suzanne and white wine for Cindy, progressing over the course of the evening to mild or moderate intoxication. It would finish with them sitting on a couch and watching one of several television shows before calling it a night.

When the therapist, after helping Suzanne and Cindy describe the totality of their constricted lifestyle, suggested that they as a couple consider being sober for a period, Cindy said yes, but Suzanne was hesitant. That was not hard to understand given Suzanne's longstanding reliance on alcohol for psychological reasons. The therapist asked them to think about the possibility of sobriety for a couple of weeks before their next session. On returning, they both said that after many talks, they were willing to pursue this advice and recognized that drinking itself had become a serious problem. But they also said they had no idea—other than sheer willpower—about how to rid their lifestyles of alcohol for any length of time.

A COMMON DILEMMA

All of these couples shared a common dilemma. On the one hand, they'd all come to the realization that drinking was exerting a significant and negative impact on their relationships. In effect, it was "hollowing out" their relationships. They'd also concluded that sobriety was a good idea—even for a while. At the same time, they didn't know how to go about achieving this goal, about what barriers they should expect to encounter or how to deal with them. They also had some trepidations—personally and in terms of their social networks—as to how this decision would be received by the people in their lives.

Make no mistake about it—the journey to sobriety can be complicated and challenging, but the information in this book can help. The issues that couples who find themselves drinking too much have, until now, received very little attention. This book corrects that. As we move forward, we will explore how couples caught in this conundrum can find their way out and move from *shared misery* to *sober love*.

Chapter 4

WHAT IT TAKES

ONCE YOU HAVE TAKEN the time together to do an honest assessment of where each of you falls on the drinking spectrum, the next step is to decide what, in anything, you want to do next as a couple. Here are some suggestions for starting the discussion:

- On a scale of 1 (least) to 10 (most), how motivated are each of you, today, to become a sober couple?
- If there is a significant discrepancy between your motivational ratings (three or more), what might it take to bring you closer together?
- Finally, if one of you is further along on the spectrum than the other, can you nevertheless support one another in seeking to be a sober couple?

Let's assume that each of you falls somewhere between the "mild" and "moderate" range on the drinking spectrum—maybe a bit more toward moderate. This means that you regularly drink more than the "low-risk" range defined by experts, but less than the "severe" range (what is sometimes defined as alcoholism). In addition, you recognize that drinking has affected you both as individuals and as a couple. If that is the case, now is a good time for you to face the following decisions:

- What should be your goal?
- What tools will you need to succeed?

We need to explore each of these questions in turn. But first let's look at another example.

One of the challenges to becoming a sober couple is encountering the people, places, and routines associated with drinking, including their social network, family, and sometimes even coworkers and colleagues. Couples are often reluctant to address these situations—let alone change them—in part because they do not want to offend or alienate friends or family members. They may fear losing their social network, becoming outcasts by defying a family or friendship culture, or just seeming "abnormal" in the context of a drinking culture.

HELEN AND TED

Helen, age 65, and her husband Ted, 67, had sold their New England home two years earlier and moved south to a comfortable retirement community. They loved the warm weather, as well as the company that was available at the clubhouse and pools of their gated senior community.

Both Ted and Helen had long enjoyed an afternoon cocktail, a ritual that long preceded retirement. On rare occasions they might have two, but no more than that. But since moving and getting involved in the new community, their drinking had steadily increased, and they had gradually moved along the drinking spectrum. Now, between regular clubhouse gatherings and frequent informal social engagements at their home and others', they were both consuming 15 or more cocktails every week. Helen and Ted were unaware that they were part of an aging demographic with the greatest increase in drinking over the past decade or more. This group—people age 60 and older—has much higher rates of heavy drinking, possibly as a consequence of increased isolation due to divorce, widowhood, and separation from extended family.

Although not alcoholics, Ted and Helen's level of drinking was substantially more than what is considered "low-risk drinking" by national standards. In fact, their level of drinking put them in the "excessive drinking" category, or what would qualify as at least a mild alcohol use disorder. But because they had slid into this category slowly over a year or more, and partly by becoming accustomed to the drinking norms of their new community, they were not cognizant of being in any danger. In short, they did not see the connection between their changing drinking pattern and its consequences. But Helen and Ted did face consequences, some apparent and others lurking beneath the surface.

Helen was a breast cancer survivor, having been cancer-free for five years. Still, she had a family history of cancer, including her mother and sister, plus an aunt who died from cancer. Drinking as much as she did now put her at risk for cancer to recur, either in a breast or elsewhere. For his part, Ted had undergone surgery to have two stents installed in his heart. He was the first to experience symptoms that related to his increased drinking. The first of these was insomnia. He'd never had trouble sleeping soundly, but over the past six months he'd found himself unable to sleep through the night. He'd wake up in the wee hours and toss and turn, unable to get back to sleep. This led to him being groggy and lethargic the next day. Helen mentioned that alcohol could be to blame, but Ted dismissed it as a sign of aging. He used the same attribution to explain the fact that he'd begun to experience difficulty maintaining an erection on the increasingly rare occasions when they attempted to have sex.

But then Ted experienced tightness in his chest, which motivated him to see a doctor. After a thorough assessment (including taking a history of Ted's drinking as well as an echocardiogram), the doctor informed Ted that his symptoms were an early sign of a potential return of the circulatory problem that had led to the stents, and that drinking could be a contributing factor. He strongly advised Ted to either stop drinking altogether or limit himself to no more than five cocktails per week. He also scheduled a follow-up for three months later.

This presented both Helen and Ted with a challenge. Following the doctor's advice would mean significant changes in terms of people, places, and routines. If Ted were to try to limit himself to no more than five drinks a week, what would that mean for Helen? On the one hand, unlike Ted, she was not experiencing any alarming physical symptoms; on the other hand, she knew from reading as well as talking with friends and family that drinking did increase her risk for a recurrence of cancer. She knew women who'd had just such recurrences. Making changes would mean altering their clubhouse and home gathering activities. That was one thing, but what about their long-standing routine of daily afternoon cocktails?

Despite having a strong and long marriage, Helen had a hard time coming to terms with Ted's newly recommended limitation. For one thing, both her and Ted's drinking had steadily increased over the past year, and in truth she'd found herself getting used to it—even looking forward to it. She expressed both dismay and reluctance about the idea of limiting their social contacts, almost all of which included drinking.

At first, Ted tried reassuring Helen that it would be okay with him if he had only the five drinks a week, either at home or at a social gathering, while she could have as many as she wanted. Naturally, that left open the issue of their new social network. What should they do? And what should they say? Ted suggested they simply step up and share the results of Ted's exam as well as his doctor's advice. That could mean spending less time at the clubhouse or foregoing some activities that included drinking, if that's what it took to help Ted stick to the limit. It could mean seriously curtailing their social life.

When they decided to be honest and share Ted's medical concern, their new social circle mostly accepted him drinking less (actually, a lot less, and often not at all), but they did not seem to see any need to cut down on their own drinking, which Ted and Helen now realized was quite a bit more than the low-risk level. Helen admitted that she found this situation frustrating, as she did not really want to curtail their newfound social life. She would want to drink on these occasions even while being supportive of Ted's efforts to cut back. She admitted that she thought the stress of walking this line sometimes came out in the form of irritability on her part.

Six weeks later, Ted had substantially reduced his alcohol consumption but was still significantly beyond the five-drink limit. In fact, there were several social occasions when he'd gone way over his limit. He'd avoided talking to Helen about his struggle, but she sensed it. As his follow-up appointment approached, Ted felt an obligation to finally bring it into the open.

Helen's initial reaction was not all that positive. She said that she had limited herself to a single cocktail a day at home and had assumed (hoped) that Ted would just follow the doctor's advice. Ted responded that he was aware of what Helen was doing, but it was just too difficult for him to completely break a routine that had been such a central part of their lives for so many years, as well as to stay sober at social gatherings. He said he now believed they both needed to make a change if he was to reliably reduce his drinking. Helen said she needed some time to think about it, and Ted agreed to give her the space to do so.

They settled on two changes. First, they agreed that, three days a week, they would substitute a walk along the community's many walking paths for their usual afternoon cocktails. As a compromise, they also agreed that Helen could indulge in a cocktail in another part of the condo while Ted picked up on his long-standing interest in watching a variety of sporting events on TV in another room. That meant that they would not be sharing cocktails—or be together—as often as they were accustomed to, but they agreed that it was a necessary change.

The rule of thumb is that it takes roughly 90 days for a new habit or routine to begin to feel comfortable and replace a former routine. During this initial 90-day period, both Ted and Helen admitted that there were times they felt uncomfortable and yearned for a return to their old ritual. But because they agreed that it was important to Ted's health, they stuck with it. In time, Helen came to agree that reducing her drinking was best for her, a cancer survivor, as well.

That left the much thornier issue of their new social network and social life and its role in their drinking for Ted and Helen to solve. They decided to seek the advice of the pastor of their church, whom they had come to know as a level-headed man. When they met with the pastor, he said that while he was sympathetic to their ambivalence about giving up at least some part of the new social network they'd found in retirement, he was aware that many of the retirees in the parish drank excessively. He asked if they shared his impression, adding that Ted and Helen were not the only couple who'd increased their drinking in their senior years. Helen responded quickly that she did believe that their social network consisted of many couples who drank a lot, and she was under the impression that this had not necessarily always been the case for them, either. Ted chimed in to share his belief that at least some of the men in this social network had what he called drinking problems. Were there other couples, the pastor then asked, who seemed to drink a lot less, or even not at all? If so, how would Ted and Helen feel about shifting their social life more toward this group?

He then asked why Ted and Helen were seeking advice on this issue, and they told the pastor about Ted's medical concerns and the fact that Helen was a cancer survivor. "Have you thought about quitting altogether for a while?" the pastor asked Helen, given her family's medical history. He added that Ted's goal would no doubt be easier to achieve if they could count on each other for support. He explained that he personally knew of several other couples who'd made this decision, also based largely on health reasons. With regard to sharing the decision not to drink with others, the pastor said, "You don't need to apologize. Just say you're taking a break from drinking for health reasons."

After mulling it over for a few days, Ted and Helen decided to take the pastor's advice. They both agreed that quitting for an unspecified period might actually be less daunting than trying to negotiate all sorts of compromises, as they'd done until then.

WHAT SHOULD YOUR GOAL BE WITH RESPECT TO SOBER LOVE?

Many couples considering sober love wonder whether they should pursue a path of moderation or abstinence. As Helen and Ted's example shows, negotiating "rules" around trying to cut back is often more difficult than quitting altogether. Researchers who have studied the issue of recovery from substance use have consistently and convincingly demonstrated that moderation (sometimes called "controlled drinking") is not likely to be successful when a person's drinking falls even at the edge of the moderate zone on the drinking spectrum. (For more information on this research, see the sources in the appendix.) People who choose abstinence as their goal have much better outcomes than those who choose controlled drinking.

In fact, many people report that it is easier to quit than it is to control drinking.

Some clinicians and programs advertise controlled drinking as their goal, usually using the term "harm reduction." But the research simply doesn't support this approach for people whose drinking extends beyond the mild zone. Harm reduction may be a compassionate approach for those who are addicted to opioids and are at continual risk for overdose and death, but it does not apply as easily to drinking. It's up to readers to honestly assess the choices for themselves.

Even if one of you is further along on the spectrum, if you both fall somewhere in or close to that moderate range, sober love would be the best option in terms of your likely success. And even if one of you feels like you are more toward the mild end of the moderate section on the spectrum, quitting may be the best choice for your relationship.

HOW LONG?

Once you have decided on sober love, it is time to consider *how long* a period you will set as a goal. I recommend that couples commit to one year. If that strikes you as unrealistic, consider that building a sober lifestyle is not much different than building other aspects of a healthy lifestyle, like physical fitness or diet. Commitments like these, as rewarding as they can be, take time to bear fruit. Committing to a physical fitness program for only, say, three months is not likely to lead to significant changes in your overall health any more than signing up for six yoga sessions is likely to lead to reduced stress (whereas committing to yoga for a year has been found to do just that). The same is true for changing your eating habits: going vegetarian for 30 days is not likely to lead to any dramatic change in how a person feels.

In a similar way, sharing sobriety for three months is not long enough for a couple to realize the rewards of sober love. You and your partner will need more time to truly appreciate what your relationship, as well as the world in general, will look like through a sober lens.

WHAT DO COUPLES NEED TO SUCCEED?

To a large extent, the answer to this question involves all of the dimensions discussed in chapter 2. But couples must focus in on the most important factors that will make a difference between success and failure in becoming a sober couple.

There are three main factors to consider when a couple approaches the challenge of building a sturdy sober lifestyle: hardiness, support, and love. We can think of these factors as three legs of a stool. In order to function effectively, a stool requires not one, not two, but at least three sturdy legs. Moreover, the best stools have legs that are connected so that they support one another.

HARDINESS

Let's begin with the first factor—or "leg"—which is psychological hardiness. Also known as resilience, this personality style was first named and studied in the late 1970s. Psychologists investigated hardiness it by studying men and women who had what you could call high-stress careers (executives, police officers, teachers, military personnel). They then separated these individuals into two groups: those who were prone to being healthy, both physically and psychologically, whom they called *hardy*, versus those who were more prone to illness and mental disorders, whom they labeled *fragile*.

The researchers found some significant differences in the personality styles of these two groups, and it turns out they are relevant when it comes to looking at sober love. We call the components of hardiness the "Three C's": Commitment, Control, and Challenge.

Commitment

Psychologically hardy people are prone to making firm commitments and sticking to them. This can involve their career, their health, their personal goals and values, and so on. They do not easily abandon these commitments. For psychologically fragile individuals, in contrast, *the road to failure is paved with half-hearted commitments.* In contemplating sober love, you as a couple need to consider which of these camps you want to belong to: you either make a commitment to a period of sober living, or you make a half-hearted commitment that allows you to think of an easy way out. People who relapse from recovery to serious addiction tend to fall in the latter group. They talk themselves out of a commitment to being sober, usually by falling victim to a fantasy about being able to drink or use drugs safely. As a couple, neither of you may yet have moved into the severe range on the drinking spectrum, which is associated with true alcoholism. Nevertheless, the issue of whether you do decide to share a commitment to a significant period of sobriety (and stick to it) is important.

Control

Control is a belief that we either possess the skills necessary to keep our commitments and achieve our goals or that we can learn them. A lack of control, then, is simply not having faith in ourselves. In effect, control boils down to self-confidence, or what psychologists like to call *self-efficacy.* The purpose of this book is to guide you as a couple in anticipating and planning for the skills you will need to experience sober love. Pause here to reflect on your own self-confidence, given your past experiences in pursuing goals. Even if you experience some anxiety around self-control, rest assured that the tools provided here, combined with your own creativity and perseverance, will get you through.

Challenge

People who are psychologically hardy were found to have a belief that life is full of changes and potential challenges—in short, that life is not a smooth road. They are inclined to enjoy and be grateful for life when it is going well, but without becoming complacent. This personality style turns out to be a real asset when a person (or couple) finds themselves confronted with a challenge. Pursuing sober love will likely present you with challenges. As a couple, you will have an advantage if you accept this reality and prepare for it. By doing so, you will be much less apt to suffer from any debilitating anxiety, and much less likely to feel helpless and abandon your commitment.

SUPPORT

Success at becoming a sober couple requires a commitment, but good intentions alone, as most of us know from experience, are often not enough to achieve a major change in our lifestyles. That brings us to the second leg on the stool. The reality is, sober couples face having to finds ways to live and thrive in a drinking culture. They may find themselves feeling isolated, just as individuals whose social network normalizes and supports drinking can find themselves pretty much alone in pursuing a goal of sobriety.

In order to bolster their chances of realizing their respective goals, both individuals and couples are faced with a critical choice: either build a social network that supports being sober, or identify such a social network and find a way to utilize its support in ways that they find comfortable. One major source of such support are the many recovery fellowships that promote sobriety through social support.

The fellowship that most often comes to mind is Alcoholics Anonymous, because it is so ubiquitous. AA meetings are easily found through its website, www.AA.org. In 2020, AA conducted a member survey that counted more than 2 million AA members and over 120,000 AA groups in 180 countries—likely conservative estimates, as AA does not require groups to report their membership.

Some people, even professionals, are skeptical of AA, regarding it as a cult or confusing it with a religion (it is neither). But much research has been conducted on AA over the past 20 years. After rigorously evaluating 35 studies involving more than 10,000 participants, researchers at Harvard and Stanford concluded that AA was more effective in promoting sobriety than alternative approaches such as cognitive behavioral therapy or psychotherapy.

As ubiquitous as AA is, it is not the only place couples can turn for support. Couples—or even individuals within a couple—should consider availing themselves of AA or another fellowship to find support for sober living. There they will find people of a like mind, who care about one another and whose collective goal is to support one another. They also share a common belief that being a sober individual or couple leads to a lifestyle that is better than the drinking life.

Even though psychotherapy alone is not as effective as AA in promoting sobriety, roughly 40% of AA members report pursuing therapy in addition to attending AA. Moreover, researchers have found that the combination of AA and therapy is the most powerful predictor of long-term sobriety. This makes sense, as many AA members elect to utilize the fellowship to support being sober, with concurrent therapy to help with other issues, including those that may have contributed to their drinking in the first place. That was true for many of the couples highlighted in this book.

LOVE

There is a third powerful factor that plays a role in terms of what you will need to succeed as a couple, and that is *love*. Yes, love. That is the third leg on the stool. In order to succeed in achieving the goal of becoming a sober couple, you must have the capacity and willingness to care not just about yourself as an individual, but also about your partner and your relationship. You must be willing to commit to shared sobriety—sober love—for a determined period. Without that shared commitment, and without recognizing your relationship as that "third entity" that has a life of its own and connects you to your partner, you may find yourselves working at cross purposes, and end up experiencing more conflict than compatibility.

MOVING FORWARD

As you move forward together toward sober love, keep in mind both the level of commitment you are willing to make, as well as how you can bring the Three C's to bear on realizing it. When you find yourselves approaching your goal, that will be the time to step back and assess how far you have come together. Then decide as a couple whether to move forward with sober love.

Chapter 5

A NEW IDENTITY

The Sober Couple

EVERY PERSON MUST PASS THROUGH various developmental stages in order to eventually form and then embrace an identity. The psychologist Eric Erikson wrote about this process in his book *Identity: Youth and Crisis.* You can ask yourself the following questions to get to the heart of your identity:

- What are my physical and intellectual strengths and limitations?
- What are my social strengths and limitations?
- What are my greatest interests? Am I so passionately interested in something that I willingly spend time on it?
- What are my values? Whom do I admire, and what do I stand for?
- What are my goals?
- What does my future look like? Are my options limited, and if so, how and why?

The crucible in which our identity forms consists of the culture we live in, our family, our social network, and our personal experiences. Together, these things give us that sense of who we are, what is important to us, and what our potential is. As teens, our social network includes our peers, including those we identify with and seek out. It also includes those we are not drawn to or who reject us. Self-esteem depends on finding a peer group where a teen feels accepted and successful—a personal niche. High schools are full of such groups, but not all of them contribute to a healthy identity. At this stage of life, teens might find themselves drawn to groups known not for academic success, athletic prowess, or artistic or writing talent, but rather primarily for being outcasts that exhibit antisocial behavior or use drugs or alcohol.

As for where drinking fits into our identity, the surrounding drinking culture, personal experiences, family, and more clearly play a role in whether a person regards drinking as normal and therefore a part of who they are. For most people in our culture, drinking ends up being part of their identity. But that may be starting to change; hence this book.

CHANGE: IDENTITY AND EPIPHANY

Once formed—typically during adolescence and young adulthood—our identity tends to crystallize and become a self-fulfilling prophecy, unless some experience comes along to alter that identity. We call such experiences *epiphanies.* Dictionary.com describes one popular way of looking at epiphanies:

> *A sudden, intuitive perception of or insight into the reality or essential meaning of something, usually initiated by some simple, homely, or commonplace occurrence or experience.*

In other words, an epiphany can be triggered by something that from the outside appears relatively trivial. As an example, Jack, a man in his mid-twenties working his first job after college, met with his supervisor for a six-month performance evaluation. At the time, Jack held an entry-level position in the customer service division of an engineering firm. The supervisor, an older and experienced man whom the young man respected, said, "Jack, you're a bright and talented young man, and you can definitely handle this job. But there's one thing I've noticed about you, and that is that in my opinion you don't put out 100% of what you're capable of."

That comment proved to be life-changing for Jack. It stuck with him, in part, he said, because deep down he knew it was true, and that was because Jack was not passionate about the current career path he was on. Two years later, he changed course, returned to graduate school, and eventually became an environmental engineer doing groundbreaking work in green energy.

Here's another definition, from Merriam-Webster:

Generally the term is used to describe a scientific breakthrough or a religious or philosophical discovery, but it can apply in any situation in which an enlightening realization allows a problem or situation to be understood from a new and deeper perspective.

This definition implies that an epiphany can occur as a dramatic event, and indeed it sometimes is. Here are a couple of examples of people whose identity was changed as a result of a dramatic epiphany.

Marsha Linehan is a psychologist who created a treatment for something called borderline personality disorder, or BPD. Women who suffer from BPD have low self-esteem to the point of hating themselves, and they often engage in self-harm, such as cutting, substance misuse, and eating disorders. Linehan herself states that she suffered from BPD as a girl and young woman, including cutting and burning herself with cigarettes, to the extent of having to be restrained as a patient in a psychiatric hospital. Later, after leaving the hospital but still deeply unhappy with herself, she was in her early twenties, separated from her family, living at the YWCA (Young

Women's Christian Association), and working as a clerk. Then she had an epiphany.

She moved into another Y, found a job as a clerk in an insurance company, started taking night classes at Loyola University—and prayed, often, at a chapel in the Cenacle Retreat Center.

"One night I was kneeling in there, looking up at the cross, and the whole place became gold—and suddenly I felt something coming toward me. It was this shimmering experience, and I just ran back to my room and said, 'I love myself.' It was the first time I remember talking to myself in the first person. I felt transformed."

The high lasted about a year, before the feelings of devastation returned in the wake of a romance that ended. But something was different. She could now weather her emotional storms without cutting or otherwise harming herself.

Marsha went on to study psychology, earned a doctorate, and developed a treatment approach that has since helped many women caught up in the same quagmire of self-hatred.

Malcolm X, the one-time radical but later civil rights leader, started out as a teen leading a life of crime, and he was eventually incarcerated. He described himself at that time as someone who was intensely angry and alienated, and who held white people responsible for the prejudice that he believed was at the root of his and other Black people's persecution. That anger formed the core of his initial identity. But Malcolm X, too, ended up being profoundly affected by an epiphany. It occurred after leaving prison and traveling abroad as a member of his new religion, Islam, and it happened this way:

In Saudi Arabia, Malcolm experienced what amounted to his second life-changing epiphany as he accomplished the hajj, or pilgrimage to Mecca, and discovered an authentic Islam of universal respect and brotherhood. The experience changed Malcolm's worldview. Gone was the belief in White people as exclusively evil. Gone was the call for Black separatism. His voyage to Mecca helped him discover the atoning power of Islam as a means to unity as well as self-respect: "In my thirty-nine years on this earth," he would write in his autobiography, "the Holy City of Mecca had been the first time I had ever stood before the Creator of All and felt like a complete human being."

You might say that these two epiphanies took place in a spiritual context. They were life-changing because the result was a new identity for both Linehan and Malcolm X. The subject of this book involves an epiphany, one that is associated with a profound shift in identity, not just for individuals but in this case for a couple. It represents a major change in that sense of who they are: that being a sober couple might just be better than being a drinking couple.

Not all epiphanies are as dramatic as the two examples above, and not all are associated with what you might call a spiritual awakening. For many of us, an epiphany tends to come to us gradually, as it did for Jack, whose ultimate decision to change careers evolved over a period of two years. However it occurs, the end result, as the definitions and experiences point out, is a significant insight, a new way of looking at yourself—who you are—and the direction you choose to pursue. This applies to individuals as well as couples, since the core of any relationship is a shared identity.

EPIPHANY AND DRINKING

Make no mistake about it—epiphanies and any resulting changes in identity are often far-reaching, affecting many aspects of a person's life. Yet all who have experienced an epiphany and followed the path they now saw before them say that it was worthwhile. That is true for couples as well as individuals, as many of the examples later in this chapter will show.

The epiphany about drinking may come slowly, and not until individuals and couples devote a lot of time and energy trying to hold on to their identity as drinkers, an identity society often tells us is "normal." Often the efforts to keep drinking in their lives include things like:

- Counting drinks
- Limiting times or places for drinking (weekends, Friday happy hours, sports bars)
- Switching brands of types of liquor (wine only, beer only, hard cider only, etc.)
- Quitting for a week

These strategies might work for someone who truly believes they fall into the low-risk range of the drinking spectrum and wish to avoid sliding deeper into the spectrum. But for those who find themselves deep into the mild zone, or even the moderate zone, such efforts usually prove fruitless. Nevertheless, drinkers may persist with them for some time before deciding they are ready to try sobriety.

What kind of epiphany do people usually experience when it comes to drinking and the part it plays in their identity? One way to look at it is to consider the way recovery fellowships define this insight. There are a number of such fellowships, and their memberships are growing. What they share is a different perspective on drinking and the role they see it playing in a person's identity. Here, for example, is what *Alcoholics Anonymous*, the largest and most pervasive fellowship, has to say about it, in the first of their 12 Steps:

We admitted we were powerless over alcohol, that our lives had become unmanageable.

Readers of this book may not agree that drinking has made their lives "unmanageable." But many couples in the moderate zone on the drinking spectrum might relate to a statement like this:

We admitted to ourselves and each other that our relationship has gradually "hollowed out" as a result of drinking.

Another fellowship, *Women for Sobriety* (WFS), describes the insight or epiphany this way:

WFS believes that having a life-threatening problem with alcohol and/or other drug use is not a moral weakness, it is the symptom of a serious disorder which demands rigorous attention to healing. WFS Acceptance Statement #1: I have a life-threatening problem that once had me.

I now take charge of my life and my well-being. I accept the responsibility.

A third fellowship, *SMART Recovery*, has this to say:

Self-Management and Recovery Training (SMART) is a global community of mutual-support groups. At meetings, participants help one another resolve problems with any addiction (to drugs or alcohol or to activities such as gambling or over-eating). Participants find and develop the power within themselves to change and lead fulfilling and balanced lives guided by our science-based and sensible 4-Point Program.

Meanwhile, the fellowship *Secular AA* offers this perspective:

Our mission is to assure suffering alcoholics that they can find sobriety in Alcoholics Anonymous without having to accept anyone else's beliefs or deny their own. Secular AA does not endorse or oppose any form of religion or belief system and operates in accordance with the Third Tradition of the Alcoholics Anonymous Program: "the only requirement for AA membership is a desire to stop drinking."

The Red Road to Wellbriety is rooted in Native American culture:

The Red Road is an abstinence-based fellowship that combines the 12 step program of AA with Native American cultural beliefs. It is a holistic healing journey based on Lakota/Nakota/Dakota world views. Wellbriety has principles that it couples with the 12 Steps: Honesty, Hope, Faith, Courage, Integrity, Willingness, Humility, Justice Forgiveness, Perseverance, Spiritual Awareness and Service.

Finally, a recently developed fellowship directed specifically at couples is called *Recovering Couples Anonymous*. It describes itself this way:

RCA is open to all committed adult couples seeking to create or restore a caring, committed, and intimate monogamous relationship regardless of age, sexual orientation, gender identification, religious background, culture, race, class, national origin, physical or mental challenge, or political affiliation. Although there is no organizational affiliation between Alcoholics Anonymous and our fellowship, we are based on the principles of AA.

Fellowships like these (and there are others) are all based on the idea that an individual (or couple) can choose to pursue a new identity—as a sober individual or couple—without shame and with the expectation that doing so will lead to a more satisfying life. They rely on a shared insight: an epiphany that a life without drinking could be better.

Keep in mind that an individual or couple does not need to conclude that either or both of them fall on the extreme or severe range on the drinking spectrum to join a recovery fellowship. On the contrary, all these groups exist for the sole purpose of supporting their members in the goal of pursuing a sober lifestyle. AA, for example, requires of its members only that they desire to stop drinking. Couples need not disclose a diagnosis in order to avail themselves of the ongoing support that fellowships like AA provide. Indeed, many of my clients have shared how helpful participating in a fellowship, either in person or online, helped reinforce their decision to pursue a sober lifestyle. For them, it is akin to finding an oasis amid the drinking culture. All of these fellowships offer a pathway to that lifestyle.

SOBER LIVING AND PERSONAL RENEWAL

A central point of this book has to do with the gradual effects that drinking has on an individual's (and by extension a couple's) overall lifestyle. The further along the drinking spectrum an individual or couple finds themselves, the more negative those effects will be on health, intimacy, relationships, goals, and interests. In addition to embracing mutual support as a means of pursuing a sober lifestyle, the programs offered by recovery fellowships acknowledge this harm and seek to address it. Women for Sobriety, for example, addresses the emotional health of its members: "To overcome substance use disorders, women must address their real needs—those for an increased sense of self-value, self-worth, and self-efficacy. The WFS New Life Program is specifically designed to fit these emotional needs of women."

Many recovery fellowships—which are now, thanks in part to the Internet, more available than ever—have as their focus the whole health of the whole person. They underscore the reality that choosing a sober lifestyle is indeed choosing "a new life."

KURT AND MONICA

Kurt, a successful professional engineer, started drinking at around age 12 and had a history of not being able to control it. Both his father and paternal grandfather were what Kurt called "functional alcoholics," meaning primarily that they rarely if ever missed a day of work because of their drinking. But as Kurt pointed out, that did not mean they were functional parents. Rather, both were essentially absentee fathers.

Kurt admitted that he'd tried to limit his drinking "more times than I can count," yet each attempt had promptly led to failure. In other words, every time he drank, he'd get drunk. But Kurt clung to the idea that there were "three doors" to choose from: "door number one" was drinking without limit, "door number two" was abstinence, and "door number three" (which he preferred) was "controlled" drinking.

Now 40 and never married, Kurt had recently begun to experience pain when swallowing. Then one evening when he and his girlfriend Monica were out to dinner, he thought he might actually choke when he tried to swallow. Alarmed, Monica insisted he contact his doctor's answering service immediately.

The next day Kurt met with his doctor, who referred him to a specialist who ran some tests. The specialist advised Kurt that it seemed his esophagus was chronically irritated and that it could be a precursor to cancer. He also asked Kurt about his drinking. Despite this ominous warning, Kurt continued to flirt for some time with what he called "the third door." He saw a counselor and explained that he believed he could limit himself to no more than two drinks per day. That lasted one week. The counselor then asked if Kurt had ever considered looking into medication, a fellowship like AA, or both. Kurt replied that he'd once been admitted to a medical detox unit for four days in his early thirties—the result of having been intoxicated while in the field on an assignment—and had gotten the same advice, but he had not followed through owing to his stubborn belief that he could control his drinking.

Meanwhile, Monica was well aware of Kurt's heavy drinking when they were together. What she was not aware of was that he also drank when they were not together—for example, after dropping her off at home after a date. She followed up with Kurt regarding the disturbing event at dinner and asked what the doctors had said. Kurt decided to be honest with Monica and tell his story, including his drinking history, his belief in moderation, and even his experience with detox. He told Monica he felt ashamed, as if he was not a "normal" person because of his drinking.

Kurt's decision to come clean also opened a door for Monica. She explained that she also had a history of excessive drinking, though somewhat different from Kurt's. Rather than drinking heavily more or less continuously, Monica had a history of binge drinking, typically when she spent time with a certain group of women friends or went to a party. At home she drank much less, though she confessed that she did have a couple of glasses of wine most nights after work. She'd been able to keep this from Kurt because she did not see him in situations where she drank a lot. This had been her pattern for several years now, however, and she was not happy about it. Each time, she said, it took her longer to recover from the lethargy and general malaise that came with being hungover. Even so, she'd found it difficult to come to terms with the alternative, which would mean either not drinking when she was with her friends or avoiding those social occasions altogether.

With respect to the drinking spectrum, Monica fell somewhere in the middle of the mild zone. Kurt, however, certainly was beyond that, most likely somewhere in the middle of the moderate zone if not further along given his history of not being able to moderate his use.

Monica asked Kurt what he thought of the idea of them both giving sobriety a try. She had a friend, she said, who had decided to take a break from drinking and attended meetings of a support group called Women for Sobriety. Monica had looked it up and read some of its materials. Her friend had made that decision as the result of an insight (or epiphany) she had after the last time she'd woken up groggy after a night of heaving drinking. She realized if she continued on her current course, she could very well end up like her ailing mother, who also had a binge drinking problem that the family never faced up to. Now Monica was thinking of trying out a couple of online WFS meetings.

After hearing Monica out, Kurt spoke with his counselor about it. The counselor then simply asked, "How many times do you want to keep trying to walk through that imaginary third door?" He added that Kurt's medical consequences were serious and gave him some information about a fellowship called SMART Recovery, suggesting he check it out.

The next week, when Kurt and Monica had a dinner date, she told him in advance that she would not be drinking. Then she came out and asked him how he would feel if they both decided to not drink, perhaps for the next six months, to see what life looked like at that point. She said she believed that both of them could benefit from a break from alcohol. She valued their relationship, she said, but feared that drinking could potentially poison it.

This time Kurt did not order any drinks, but said he'd need to think about Monica's suggestion. The next day he called to say that he was on board with her idea, though he added that he needed to talk with his doctor and his counselor, as he believed, in his words, that he would need more than good intentions and Monica's support to succeed.

TAKING STOCK

As you and your partner consider the insights offered by Kurt and Monica's example and the potential benefits of recovery fellowships, the following questions can help start a discussion of your potential new identity as a sober couple:

- Where do you, both as individuals and as a couple, fall on the drinking spectrum?
- Has your drinking moved further along the drinking spectrum over time?
- What role does drinking play in your lives, and how much is it part of your identity as a couple?
- Has drinking hollowed out your relationship in any way over time?
- How have you tried to change your drinking habits or to drink less? How has this worked out?
- Overall, how satisfied are you now with your drinking life?
- Can you imagine any ways in which a sober relationship could be better?
- Do you have any reservations about becoming a sober couple?

Chapter 6

BREAKING FREE AND
MOVING FORWARD

MICHAEL AND CLYDE

Michael and Clyde had been married for four years and together for ten. Michael was a successful personal trainer with his own studio, and Clyde was an insurance executive. When they first met, they enjoyed the busy city life, including visiting new museum exhibits, eating at trendy restaurants, attending the theatre, and working out together at a nearby fitness center—all of this interspersed with occasional weekends spent at inns in the country. They also enjoyed an active social life.

At the time they decided to seek counseling, both were drinking at what Clyde described as a "pretty heavy" level. His drinking had progressed gradually over a period of several years, to the point where he was now drinking a bottle of wine every day, starting when he got home from the office (or at lunchtime on weekends). Meanwhile, Michael preferred whiskey sour cocktails, drinking at least two each weekday evening and more on weekends. It was relatively easy for them to drink that much if not more given their social circle as well as the fact that they had become more or less what Michael described as "drinking buddies."

Both Michael and Clyde had experienced negative consequences of drinking—some more obvious than others. Clyde, for example, had put on weight that he found virtually impossible to lose. The fact that they rarely went to the fitness center anymore didn't help matters. In addition, his family had a history of alcoholism, and his father, a loud and obnoxious alcoholic that the family was ashamed of, had died at a relatively young age of a heart attack that Clyde was certain was attributed to his heavy drinking. Understandably, that thought, along with some anxiety, lingered in the back of Clyde's mind.

For his part, Michael felt that his stamina had decreased significantly over time. In addition, he felt some shame in being a professional trainer who had once exercised regularly and was careful with his diet but now consumed at least two cocktails every day. Like Clyde, he had put on some pounds. He was aware, too, that the number of mornings he'd wake up feeling hungover was starting to pile up. Recently, he'd taken a nasty fall in the house while under the influence and had had to suspend his practice for ten days while a sprained shoulder healed.

Interestingly, what motivated this couple to take a closer look at their drinking and see a counselor was not these obvious consequences, but some good friends. One of the couples they knew well had recently gone public in declaring that they'd decided to get sober together. They even jokingly referred to the decision as "coming out of the closet" with their drinking. And while they'd chosen somewhat different paths, both were committed to not drinking. One had decided to meet with his physician and explain the issue. The doctor prescribed naltrexone, a medication known to help reduce cravings for alcohol, and recommended counseling as well. The other decided on another option that involved participating in online meetings of a fellowship called Secular AA. That fellowship, like AA, supports sobriety but does not make any mention of God or advocate for any religious belief. Ironically, although Bill Wilson, the founder of AA, was himself an avowed agnostic, and while AA itself is not affiliated with any religion, some people feel uncomfortable with its inclusion of the word God in several of the 12 Steps. In any case, this friend felt comfortable in these meetings, which included some members of the lesbian, gay, bisexual, transexual, and queer (LGBTQ) community, and the couple supported each other in their respective paths to their shared goal of sobriety.

SEPARATE BUT TOGETHER

Michael and Clyde's situation brings up an important issue, which is how they design their respective and shared recovery programs. Do they both need to select the same recovery fellowship? Do they need to attend meetings together, or can they each choose one or more to attend separately? In my experience, a couple's recovery plans do not need to be clones of one another as long as they are pursuing the same goal. Sharing their experiences in meetings does not necessarily mean having to attend the same meetings, with the caveat that they respect one another's choices. In other words, they can pursue the same goal together, but to some degree each will follow their own path to sobriety. Such an approach will avoid any need for conflict regarding the "best" pathway, as it recognizes that there are many pathways to the same shared end: sober love.

SHARED SECRETS

Clyde and Michael were able to be honest about their drinking and how it had progressively affected them as individuals and as a couple. Once they were willing to look back objectively on it, they agreed that in a sense they had conspired to avoid facing those consequences. Clyde labeled it as "our shared secret," while Michael described the relationship as having evolved into "drinking buddies."

But Michael and Clyde had avoided talking about another issue: sex. During counseling, Michael was the one more willing to talk about that, as he admitted he was also the more frustrated one. But whenever he had brought it up over the past couple of years, Michael's response was the same: "This is not a good time to talk about this. I'm really busy and stressed at work."

Asked to describe the current status of their sexual relationship, Michael was direct: "Very routine and brief. Bordering on boring. I'd call it 'plain vanilla' now, when it used to be very exciting." That response made Clyde visibly uncomfortable, yet he didn't deny the truth in what Michael was saying.

THE HOLLOWING

In chapter 5, we discussed how drinking can hollow out a relationship, a situation that definitely applied to Michael and Clyde. Figure 6.1 depicts how the overall relationship exists alongside the partners within it. It shows Michael and Clyde as individuals, with the overlapping part representing their relationship.

In a healthy relationship, this overlapping part is substantial, representing the partners' shared commitment to one another. It also represents those factors that bind a couple together. Another way to think of this is that the relationship between partners has a life of its own, to which they both contribute. That life includes shared values,

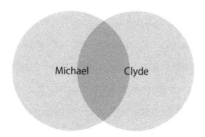

FIGURE 6.1

Where their identities overlap, Michael and Clyde's relationship exists as a third party, represented here as a Venn diagram. Their relationship can grow or wither depending on how much priority they give it.

shared goals, shared social networks, shared interests, and shared pleasures. It does not imply that a couple like Clyde and Michael have no individual interests, just that in a healthy relationship there is some significant common ground. This had certainly been true for Michael and Clyde at the outset of their relationship.

What typically happens when a couple slips along the drinking spectrum from low-risk use into the mild or moderate zones is that this shared space in the diagram gradually shrinks. In terms of what you read earlier, as the couple's "relationship" with drinking grows, the areas of common interest gradually shrink, and the relationship slowly gets hollowed out and withers. This was true for Clyde and Michael. For example, Michael noted that he and Clyde had gradually devoted less and less time together tending to the flower gardens that they once took great pride in and got lots of compliments about. There was also the gradual decline in the frequency that they walked together around their neighborhood, visited a museum, attended a theatre show, or sought out a new restaurant. It had been quite a while since they last enjoyed a weekend jaunt to a country inn. And, of course, there was the deterioration of their sex life.

There was more hollowing out, and it too had progressed gradually. For instance, they both admitted that their daily routine had shrunk, so that upon getting home after work, the first thing each would do was to have a drink and, shortly after, another. They described this as a "habit" that had become ingrained in their relationship, and one effect it had was that they found themselves spending less time sitting on their porch and sharing the days' activities and events, an activity that once was a central part of their routine. Instead, now they sat in separate lounges in front of the television and watched the news (and drank), without much conversation between them. Taken together, all of the above added up to some significant hollowing out of this once-solid relationship.

Can you identify with this process in your own relationship? Can you name some activities or interests that once constituted the common ground that bound you together but have gradually withered? Would you be interested in recovering that part of your relationship?

AMBIVALENCE

When their counselor asked them if they could relate to the idea of being *ambivalent* about the extent of their drinking and the need to do something about it, Clyde and Michael both nodded. Such ambivalence is common in both individuals and couples. It reflects a hesitance to confront the need for a change. People are often inclined to ask, *Are things really that bad?* or *Do we really need to change?* You and your partner might do well to ask yourselves these questions:

- Are we focused on mixed feelings (ambivalence) about our drinking, minimizing how it has affected our relationship?
- If so, does it just reflect our reluctance to face up to the reality of needing to make a change?

Ambivalence is not limited to this issue of sober love. In fact, ambivalence often rears its head whenever someone contemplates making a significant change in their lives—accepting a new job offer, for example, or selling a house in order to move. In such instances we often hesitate to take such a leap. We hesitate because while we know what we have, we're not sure exactly what things will look like after we make the change. Ambivalence is colored by this dynamic of a reluctance to let go of what we have now versus what we are looking for.

Ambivalence, then, reflects a hesitation to give up whatever positives we see in our current situation. It's hard to see what the positives might be if we were to exchange the status quo for a significant change. That was true for Michael, who admitted that despite the consequences to himself and his relationship with Clyde, he found himself nostalgic at times for "the good old days" when he could enjoy the buzz he'd get from sipping a whiskey sour (or two or three) while relaxing on their back porch. He also admitted that he sometimes liked to believe that his drinking could return to a scenario where he had but a single drink, though on another level he knew that he'd never really be able to limit himself to one.

SHAME

Another lesson we can draw from Michael and Clyde has to do with that issue of *shame*, which Michael experienced and often plays an important if unrecognized role in ambivalence. This was true for Clyde much more so than Michael, who other than being somewhat embarrassed to disclose their decision to become a sober couple given his profession was more open to becoming a sober couple. In fact, he believed that it could be a plus for his personal training business, as a break from alcohol would mean a boost to his stamina.

Clyde, in contrast, expressed fear that friends might reject them—and particularly him for some reason. In their couples counseling he explored this fear, with the counselor focusing on whether Clyde could identify with feelings of shame in other circumstances. That question prompted Clyde to disclose that he felt shame as far back as adolescence. Part of this had to do with being gay in a family that was openly hostile to and ridiculing of it. Whereas Michael's family had accepted his sexual orientation without much fanfare, Clyde suffered from shame and held off disclosing his orientation until he'd graduated college—and even then, he could tell his family was unhappy about it. Ever since, visiting with his family was an uncomfortable experience, and it contributed into adulthood to his ambivalence about disclosing his sexual orientation to anyone.

Another source of shame for Clyde had to do with his boisterous, obnoxious, and alcoholic father, who had a history of losing jobs because of his behavior and unreliability. He was an embarrassment to Clyde, who as a teen avoided inviting friends to the house for fear of what they might witness. This is a kind of "shame by association" that can burden people who fear the actions of others close to them might cast a shadow of rejection on themselves as well.

In counseling, Clyde and Michael initially talked about committing to six months of sobriety, and they also discussed not disclosing their decision to friends. Clyde worried about being judged negatively—as an "alcoholic" and a "loser" like his father. But after revealing the sources of his shame, and receiving a great deal of empathy and support from both Michael and their counselor, he eventually agreed that it would probably be more awkward and difficult to try keeping their decision secret than it would be to announce their decision to become a sober couple.

IT'S COMPLICATED

The example of Michael and Clyde illustrates the complexity of why we drink, a topic discussed in chapter 2. The "causes" of their drinking, and why it had drifted into at least the mid-mild if not the moderate zone on the spectrum, were varied and included social as well as psychological factors. When contemplating becoming a sober couple, it's wise to take some time to identify the factors that may have played a role in how your drinking progressed, both individually and as a couple. These factors may not be the same for both of you, just as either one of you may be somewhat further along on the drinking spectrum. Regardless of where each partner falls on the spectrum, the critical issue at this point is where you, as a couple, want to go from here.

Chapter 7

A RECIPE FOR SUCCESS

SO FAR WE HAVE DISCUSSED the critical components of sober love, and that is what *decisions* you as a couple are willing to make. After reflecting on the drinking spectrum, determining where each of you seems to fall on it, and identifying the consequences of drinking for you as individuals and as a couple, do you see any advantages to becoming a sober couple? Does it stand to enhance your lifestyle? Can it reverse any hollowing out of your relationship?

We've already looked at the stories of some couples who took stock of how drinking had affected their relationships and decided to embrace an identity as a sober couple. The issues that their examples raise, and how they solved them, may help you make your own decisions. In the coming chapters, we will take an even deeper dive into some of the pitfalls you may encounter along the way to sober love, along with strategies to address them. But those strategies will not be of much value if you and your partner have not yet decided to take this "road less traveled" toward sobriety. The choice is yours.

WHAT WILL WE NEED TO SUCCEED?

To a large extent, the answer to this question involves all of the dimensions discussed in chapter 2. But now we will turn our attention to three particular factors that are of paramount importance. One is a psychological factor, one is a social factor, and one is an emotional factor. Think of these three factors together, like a three-legged stool that supports a resilient identity as a sober couple. In a stool, true stability requires not one, not two, but three solid legs.

THE PSYCHOLOGICAL FACTOR

As discussed in chapter 4, one hallmark of successful people is that they are capable of making firm *commitments* and sticking to them. This can involve their career, their health, their personal goals and values, and so on. They do not easily abandon these commitments; once they make a decision on a goal, they stick to it. Standing in contrast are those who are inclined to abandon commitments. As stated earlier, for this latter group, *the road to failure is paved with half-hearted commitments.* They may decide, for example, to improve their health but abandon exercise, diet, yoga, and so on after a relatively brief try. They are the quintessential New Year's Eve resolution breakers. They may decide they want to pursue more education in order to advance their career, but move so slowly that there is little progress, and they eventually drop it. And so on.

In contemplating sober love, you as a couple need to consider which of these camps you want to belong to: you either make a commitment to a significant period of sober living, or you allow yourselves to think of an easy way out. The first choice is associated with men and women who are physically and mentally robust, while the second defines people who are vulnerable to depression, anxiety, hypertension, and so on. People who relapse from recovery to addiction tend to fall into the latter group. They talk themselves out of a commitment to being sober, usually by falling victim to a fantasy about being able to drink safely. Or they abandon their goal after a single slip. As a couple, neither of you may yet have moved into the severe range on the drinking spectrum, which is associated with true alcoholism. Nevertheless, the issue of whether you do decide to share a commitment to a significant period of sobriety (and stick to it) is important.

THE SOCIAL FACTOR

Couples who want to pursue an identity as a sober couple may find that their social circle presents a challenge to pursuing a sober lifestyle. Most of their friends, family members, and coworkers may drink—some quite a bit. Being immersed in a drinking culture is not really conducive to sobriety. As a couple, you will most likely find yourselves confronting the following decision: either build a social network of your own that will support your decision, or find an existing social network that supports you and avail yourselves of its social resources.

Fellowships are just one option for such social support, as discussed in chapter 5. I recommend that couples look into one or more recovery fellowships and "try them on for size." Whichever fellowship(s) you may try, a common denominator is a group of like-minded individuals who share a goal of pursuing a sober lifestyle. Such groups offer mutual support and the shared belief that sobriety has much to offer over the drinking life.

In recent years following the COVID-19 pandemic, the Internet has aided the proliferation of recovery fellowships. While in-person fellowship meetings became scarce during the long COVID lockdown, ingenuity came into play. Today, it's possible to "shop" the Internet to explore fellowships and meetings where one or both partners might find support from people who share their goal of an alcohol-free lifestyle. The following online resources may be good places to start as you look for the right fellowship for you.

The Online Secular AA and Recovery Meetings spreadsheet is a regularly updated list of a variety of secular peer-to-peer networks, including LifeRing, SMART, Dharma Recovery/Refuge Recovery (secular Buddhism), along with CODA + Al-Anon resources. To access the spreadsheet, visit https://bit.ly/secularmeetings.

Alcoholics Anonymous offers a valuable online resource for anyone interested in exploring the growing diversity within as a source of support. See www.EverythingAA.com.

THE EMOTIONAL FACTOR

Keep in mind that there is another force that plays a role—perhaps the most important role—in terms of what you will need to succeed as a couple, and that is *love*. In addition to fostering psychological hardiness and exploring social support, you must have the capacity to care about yourselves as individuals, your partner, and your relationship (that "third party" that connects you) enough to be willing to make a firm commitment to shared sobriety. That is the essence of sober love. Without this shared commitment, you may very well find yourselves working at cross-purposes and end up experiencing more conflict than compatibility.

As Romeo and Juliet taught us, love is a powerful force. It drives us to be not only attracted to but committed to that which we love. Like an epiphany, love can alter the course of our lives. It is the opposite of hate, which repels us and motivates us to move away. We humans are wired to experience both emotions. When we find love, we work hard to keep it and will grieve losing it deeply.

Love also involves empathy, or the ability to see things from a loved one's perspective—to put ourselves in their shoes, so to speak, and thereby understand their experience and their behavior. There are times in any relationship when conflict may get in the way of our capacity to empathize. At such times it can be helpful to keep in mind the third "C" component of hardiness—challenge—which is the ability to accept the reality that life will throw us some curve balls from time to time. Relationship conflicts are a fact of life. Maintaining a positive perspective on relationships (and life in general) means also having the belief that such obstacles can be overcome and that we can move forward again.

A robust sober relationship, in this writer's opinion, is best built on that idea of the three-legged stool. It's possible to pursue a relationship on a less fortified base, but it may be less resilient. I therefore urge readers to reflect on hardiness, support, and love and have an ongoing dialogue about where they believe their relationship stands in each of these areas, and what they might do to strengthen it.

WHAT SHOULD OUR GOAL BE WITH RESPECT TO SOBER LOVE?

Regardless of whether one of you is further along on the drinking spectrum than the other, if you both fall somewhere in the moderate to severe range, quitting (sober love) is your best option. Even if one of you feels like you are more toward the mild end of the spectrum, you would be wise to consider pursuing sober love as a couple anyway.

The next thing to consider is *how long* a period of sober love should you set as a goal. Forever? Depending on where one or both of you fall on the drinking spectrum, a decision to quit once and for all may indeed be the answer. For those men and women who fall in the severe zone, support may be necessary to stay the course. Seeking the support of fellowships like those described earlier can be nothing short of a lifesaver.

For those couples whose drinking and its consequences—both to them as individuals and as a couple—fall somewhere in the mild to moderate range, I have recommended a year of living as a sober couple. Sharing sobriety for a year will lead to your being able as a couple to assess the benefits of a sober lifestyle as compared to a drinking lifestyle—in other words, to reap the rewards of sober love.

MOVING FORWARD

As you move forward together toward sober love, keep in mind both the level of commitment you are willing to make, as well as how you can bring the Three C's to bear on realizing it. When you find yourselves approaching your goal, that will be the time to step back and assess where you have come together, as compared to where you began. At that time, you need to decide together whether to move forward with sober love or to take a step backward to the lifestyle you had before.

Chapter 8

BUILDING A SOBER LIFESTYLE

Shared Pleasures

AS DRINKING PROGRESSES along the spectrum, it gradually hollows out a relationship, much like insects can gradually hollow out the trunk of a once sturdy tree. The analogy doesn't end there either, because when viewed from the outside, it may not be obvious that the tree is weak and even vulnerable to collapse. A drinking couple's relationship is much the same. To family, friends, and even colleagues and coworkers, the effects of drinking may not be apparent until it's too late. After all, how many of us have a window into the private lives of couples we know? From the outside, these couples may seem to be perfectly happy and functional, but that is only a façade that they choose to present. After all, who wishes to present themselves as dysfunctional?

Individuals and couples whose drinking has become a problem that is not readily apparent to others may be what is known as "high-functioning alcoholics." Though their drinking may not have progressed to the severe zone on the spectrum, the high-functioning alcoholic's lifestyle, relationships, and even health have likely suffered some consequences that aren't obvious to an outside observer. But to an intimate partner, the consequences to the relationship of progressive drinking become clear once someone shines a light on them. In earlier chapters, we learned about some couples who had drifted over time into at least the mild if not the moderate zone on the spectrum. It was only once they honestly assessed their drinking and the current state of their relationships—often in response to some consequence related to drinking—that they were able to move forward with sober love.

LOST PLEASURES: TAKING AN INVENTORY

One way that a couple can get in touch with just how much drinking has affected their lifestyle is to begin with an inventory. I like to call this inventory "What It Used to Be Like," borrowing from the popular 1973 film *The Way We Were*.

Perhaps the best baseline for this exercise is to think back to the early days of your relationship, or at least to a time when you both drank significantly less than you do now. Take some time to peruse the following list, and note how many of these "shared pleasures" you enjoyed together back then, as well as how often they were part of your lives:

- *Intimacy*: How much time did you spend just being together and talking, sharing your respective days' activities or notable events? How often did you chat over a meal or while taking a walk, sitting on a couch, or taking care of daily chores and routines? Did you listen to what each other had to say? How intimately did you share the details of your day-to-day lives?
- *Physical touch*: How often did you give each other hugs and kisses? Did you hold hands or snuggle in public?
- *Sex*: What was your sex life like, including making love and the run-up to actual sex (foreplay, sexual touch)? How long did sex typically last, and did you both feel satisfied when it ended? Were you "on the same page" in terms of how often you had sex? How about what sex consisted of?

- *Cooking/sharing meals*: Was this ever a part of your relationship? How often did it happen? What were your favorite meals? Did you shop for ingredients together?

- *Exploration*: Early on, couples often spend time together exploring. Did you ever stroll through parks and neighborhoods or visit interesting stores? What about hiking or biking on trails? How often did you visit local town fairs, farmers markets, or music venues?

- *Nostalgia*: Can you think of a favorite restaurant you used to enjoy regularly? What movies were your favorite? How often did you and your partner visit with good friends?

- *Adventure*: When was the last time you planned a weekend away or went on vacation, just the two of you? Have you recently visited a new restaurant or planned a major event, such as a home renovation?

- *Socializing*: How often did you spend time with friends old and new? Did you ever check out a new social event or explore a new interest together?

- *Homemaking*: Did you and your partner share outdoor activities like gardening? What about interior activities like decorating or purchasing a new piece of furniture (together), as well as tending to minor repairs around the house?

- *Culture*: Did you as a couple pursue any cultural activities, such as visiting a museum or gallery, attending an event in the community, seeing a play, or going to a concert or sporting event?

- *Other favored shared activities*: What else did you do together that helped to make up the "fabric" of your relationship?

CRYSTAL AND JAMAL

Crystal and Jamal had been married for just over ten years and had two young children—a daughter, Jenna, age 8, and a son, Jason, age 6. Their initial reason for seeking counseling had to do with frequent conflicts they were having "over just about everything," according to Crystal. While they didn't actually argue about everything, it was apparent that this marriage had been under strain for some time. The sources of the strain were not unfamiliar to their counselor: the stress and expense of having young children, having to manage their income much more closely than in their earlier days together, and maintaining a home and family while also juggling two careers. On top of that, Jenna had recently been diagnosed with attention deficit disorder, which contributed to her difficulties in school. She was working with a therapist and taking prescribed medication to treat her ADD and help her succeed in school. Meanwhile, Jason had started Cub Scouts, which involved weekly meetings in addition to activities such as working on badges. As much as they were committed to these things, they also added to the couple's list of responsibilities.

When the counselor asked the couple if they'd noticed any changes in their relationship and lifestyle over time, other than those attributable to entering the parenting stage of life, Crystal responded that—in addition to the growing list of child-centered responsibilities—Jamal had noticeably increased his beer drinking over time. She also confessed that she too had increased her drinking—in her case, white wine. At that point she was working from home, while Jamal went into the office every day. As Crystal described it, the first thing Jamal did when he got home from work was to pop a beer. And when the kids got off the school bus and walked into the house, pretty much the first thing that Crystal did was pour a glass of wine. They had their first drinks *before* preparing dinner, while supervising the kids as they changed out of school clothes, grabbed a snack, and did homework.

As the evening progressed, Crystal and Jamal would typically each indulge in at least two more drinks, and sometimes more. Whereas that had not been the case earlier in the relationship, drinking was now a virtual daily habit. This change, she admitted, along with a growing list of responsibilities, correlated with both of them seeming to get more irritable, impatient, and prone to being testy with each other. Crystal also volunteered that she was increasingly likely to go to bed right after the kids were settled in, to read or catch up with friends on social media, and then fall asleep. That was after she'd had a few glasses of wine. Needless to say, her early bedtime created a barrier to their sex life.

Crystal and Jamal were both college educated and had good jobs. Yet it was clear from the discussion with their counselor that their relationship was under stress, likely because of their lifestyle. When the counselor asked them to take home a questionnaire, one much like the inventory described above, and think about it between sessions, they returned looking less than exuberant. Crystal was the first to speak, and speak up she did, flatly saying that while she and Jamal had once enjoyed many of the things listed, the answer now, as she put it, other than drinking every night, was "pretty much a big fat zero."

Jamal and Crystal's relationship was a good example of the progressive hollowing out that drinking does to a relationship. In their case, like many others, it isn't difficult to understand. Transitioning from a couple to a family put a squeeze on their relationship, but their drinking routine, which put them both at least in the beginning of the moderate zone on the drinking spectrum, only exacerbated the stress they felt. Naturally, they had not set out to develop a shared drinking problem. Their relationship with drinking happened more or less spontaneously in response to a lifestyle that had become more crowded and stressful over time. People have turned to alcohol as a means of coping with stress for generations, so there was nothing "pathological" about Jamal and Crystal. Still, the effects of drinking—which compounded the normal strains typical of their stage in life—on the quality of their relationship were clear. Speaking to this, Crystal noted that she believed that the increased tension between her and Jamal could be attributed at least partly to the fact that their escalating drinking habits caused them both to lose some of the vitality that initially characterized their relationship. She felt, too, that the loss of this vitality had in turn contributed to their shared irritability and more frequent spats.

Jamal and Crystal decided to continue with counseling, using it to pursue two goals: becoming a sober couple a least for the foreseeable future, and working toward restoring some of those things that had brought them together and formed the bond that was the core of their marriage.

RECOVERING SHARED PLEASURES

The hollowing-out phenomenon associated with progression along the drinking spectrum tends to be so gradual as to be imperceptible, but once a couple is able to stop and assess their relationship in perspective, it becomes apparent. That was true for Crystal and Jamal. When they first met and began dating, neither of them was anything close to a daily drinker. Jamal described himself then as someone with a "full life." He devoted the bulk of his time and energy to his schooling, earning undergraduate and graduate degrees in a demanding business major. He had friends, none of which were heavy drinkers or partiers. Instead, when he wasn't working, Jamal enjoyed working out regularly, playing pickup basketball, and cycling.

Jamal's personality appealed to Crystal, who was also a responsible, hard-working type. Like Jamal, she was athletic, having played
field hockey in college, as well as social to the extent of joining a sorority. She did not indulge in drinking nearly as much as some of her
sorority sisters, though. It was their common interest in being active
that first attracted Crystal and Jamal. She too had a bike, and they
enjoyed taking long cruises through the nearby countryside, often
pausing for lunch along the way. Also into regular exercise, Crystal
often worked out with Jamal. They found that they shared a burgeon-
ing interest in cooking and eating healthy, and enjoyed doing it together. Last but not least, they had a mutual attraction that fueled a
vital sex life.

Over their two-year courtship, Jamal and Crystal found common ground in attending some sporting events at his alma mater
(basketball in particular) as well as action movies on the big screen.
Their lifestyle began to change, naturally, after their daughter was
born, and even more so after their son arrived. Still, Crystal had two
sisters who babysat on occasion, and Jamal's parents watched the
kids on special occasions like their anniversary. Even so, the couple
slowly found themselves falling into the patterns of drinking that
eventually led to their seeking counseling. Why they drank wasn't a
mystery, as the other competing responsibilities of married life and
parenthood inevitably demanded their time, energy, and resources.

Jamal and Crystal took advantage of the insight they gained
through counseling to chart a pathway forward. They understood that they could not change things overnight. As time passed
and their drinking gradually moved from the low-risk zone into the
mild and then possibly the moderate zone, they could see that much
of the energy and vitality of their relationship had dissipated. As
Crystal described it, it began with looking forward to that glass of
Chardonnay when she got home from a day at the office and while

she and Jamal tended to the kids and got dinner ready. "It relaxed me," she explained, "and I'd really looked forward to it."

Crystal was doing what humans have been doing for centuries, which was using alcohol to produce a calming effect. For those who are able to maintain a low level of use indefinitely, that effect may indeed be rewarding and associated with no significant consequences. For every one of those people, however, there are innumerable others whose alcohol consumption gradually increases. That's due to the common human capacity to develop a "tolerance" for alcohol, meaning that over time we need to drink more to produce the same effect. That's also exactly what happened to Crystal and Jamal, and in time it took its toll in the form of reduced vitality and the hollowing out of their relationship. Crystal realized that drinking was probably responsible for her earlier and earlier bedtimes, with less and less energy to spare. Their sex life also declined, which Crystal initially attributed to postpartum changes in her sex drive. Jamal tried to accept this, but he still expressed his frustration from time to time, often in the form of irritability instead of discussing the issue directly.

Their counselor gave Jamal and Crystal a list of some self-help groups and fellowships that provided support to people who wanted to stay sober. After thinking about it, they decided that it would be easier to stop drinking altogether rather than to try to cut down on their drinking. They felt they could do this together with support from their counselor.

Making use of counseling, along with a commitment to be a sober couple in the interest of improving their relationship, Jamal and Crystal made slow but steady progress toward rekindling some of the shared pleasures that once formed the bond at the core of their relationship but had been crowded out by their growing relationship with drinking. Their goal now was to start small, gradually recovering the ground that had been lost. Figure 8.1 shows a pie chart that

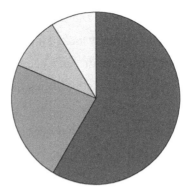

FIGURE 8.1

Jamal and Crystal's life responsibilities can be visualized as a pie chart, with some commitments requiring much more time and effort than others. A small slice of their time should be devoted to the shared pleasures they enjoy in their relationship.

can be used to visualize Jamal and Crystal's life responsibilities. They hoped that by becoming a sober couple, they could create at least a small slice of shared pleasures, the remainder being divided among all those additional things that demanded their time and commitments.

Jamal and Crystal's initial recovered shared pleasures included the following:

- Going out for dinner together once a month, relying on one of Crystal's sisters to watch the kids.
- Resuming their interest in attending college basketball games (albeit only two or three a season), with Jamal's parents doing the sitting.
- Limiting the time that they each spent on the Internet to no more than half an hour each night, thereby leaving more time for intimacy, including just sitting together for 15 or 20 minutes after the kids went to bed.
- Joining a local gym that offered childcare, and going together twice a week.

· Going to listen to live music, also once a month, eating appetizers but drinking only juice or soda.

Jamal and Crystal felt that they could manage the above, especially if they committed to being sober, and also joked with their counselor that it seemed like a "big deal" to commit that much-shared pleasure. The counselor commiserated, knowing full well how many couples in their situation struggled to carve out any quality time together. Yet that seemed as essential as any of their other commitments if their relationship was to thrive. Happily, a little over a month into these changes, they were beginning to yield positive results, including in their sex life. Crystal attributed this to two factors: spending less time in bed on the Internet, and feeling more energetic thanks to not drinking.

YOUR SHARED PLEASURES

It goes without saying that not all couples' shared pleasures will be the same. You may not share any of those that were important to Jamal and Crystal. That said, now would be a good time for you and your partner to each reflect individually on the following:

· What shared interests and activities were important to you earlier in your relationship?
· What role did those interests and activities play in what you wanted in a relationship?
· How much did these things contribute to the bond that connected you as a couple?
· Can you imagine any activities or interests you have now that you might share as a couple?

After you've had some time to think about shared pleasures, it's time to have a conversation about it, just as Crystal and Jamal did. A counselor could facilitate this conversation. It can also help to recognize how your lifestyle as a couple may have evolved over time, and how competing priorities may have squeezed out previous shared pleasures. Thinking in terms of the above pie chart can also be helpful, as it recognizes that recovering shared pleasures may mean making some room in your lifestyle while recognizing that other priorities and commitments can't be conveniently ignored. It's important to have realistic expectations, which will prevent feelings of disappointment if you look to make too many changes too soon.

It's also important to face up together to just how much drinking may have crowded out your shared pleasures over time. How did this happen? Was it just that drinking came to take up more and more time? Did drinking sap your energy, as it did for Jamal and Crystal? Did looking forward to drinking begin to take precedence over looking forward to time spent together?

Now it's time to sketch out an initial play for recovering shared pleasures. Again, keep it simple at first. On the one hand, don't make a list so long that it will be impossible to achieve, thereby leaving you feeling deflated. On the other hand, do keep in mind how much time and energy you'll gain by not drinking.

MOVING FORWARD

With this chapter we began to make some concrete inroads into living as a sober couple. Examples like Jamal and Crystal can serve as useful food for thought as you reflect on your own relationship and the changes you might consider making. If you are like most couples, you will discover that making certain changes does unleash some feelings between you that are undeniably loving and affectionate—feelings that strengthen the bond that connects you. As we move forward, we will build on this initial foundation of shared pleasures, at times focusing on removing roadblocks to sober love as well as building new structures on it.

Chapter 9

RENOVATING YOUR LIFESTYLE

HAVE YOU EVER MADE a major renovation to your life? Most people have, usually when facing some kind of transition. Often these transitions coincide with developmental change, such as going from being single to being a couple, going from being a couple to being a family, "moving up" from a smaller to a larger (or from a more modest to a more upscale) living space, "scaling down" after retirement, and so on.

DAVID AND MARION

As an example, consider one couple, David and Marion. Both had recently retired from long careers as community college professors. They had one grown daughter, an attorney who had been married to her wife for eight years and had a 3-year-old adopted daughter. They lived about an hour apart, so the family had the opportunity for fairly regular contact.

Though Marion and David had long enjoyed a list of colleagues whom they counted as friends, the reality was that much of that contact had occurred in the context of work: classes, advising, committee assignments, and the like. That was supplemented by occasional social gatherings, though in actuality these were fairly rare events. Meanwhile, several of their one-time colleagues had decided to relocate after retiring. Through the years, Marion and David's shared pleasures as a couple had consisted of board games (especially Scrabble), jigsaw puzzles, dining in fine restaurants, walking along a nearby rail trail, gardening, watching the National Geographic and public television channels, traveling once a year to visit a national park, and attending Boston Red Sox baseball games, which they did several times each season. All in all, you could say that theirs was a lifestyle rich in shared pleasures. But retirement threatened to change that lifestyle along with the loss of the collegial environment and friends as they moved away.

Shortly after retiring, Marion and David decided that now that they would be spending a lot more time at home, it would be a good idea to make some renovations that they'd always talked about but never acted on. So they hired a contractor who renovated their kitchen (they both enjoyed cooking but had long suffered with cramped space) and then expanded their backyard patio, installing a four-person hot tub next to their prized flower garden. About a year into their new retired lifestyle, however, David and Marion found themselves running into a bit of a problem.

The problem began, innocently enough, with Marion and David deciding that now that they could enjoy what seemed to them like a new home, they would entertain small groups on a more regular basis than they had up to that point—in effect, "renovating" not only their home, but also their lifestyle. They still had a large group of friends to choose from, but they limited these social occasions to no more than three other couples, so as to make them a bit more intimate and less of a fuss. Their house then quickly became a popular destination. Their remaining colleagues, much like Marion and David, proved eager to reestablish their social connections. The gatherings included cocktails or wine, along with appetizers or a light dinner.

Typically their guests would contribute something to the fare, including the drinks.

Along the way, and as their newly renovated lifestyle took hold, David and Marion (almost unconsciously) found themselves drinking considerably more than they had before. They would typically have at least three glasses of wine during social gatherings, and eventually they progressed to having a couple or more drinks most nights of the week.

Neither David nor Marion were (yet) very far along on the drinking spectrum, but they were no longer at the low-risk level. It was Marion who first noticed some consequences associated with their increased drinking, though she did not initially attribute these to drinking. They included poor sleep followed by some notable lethargy in the morning, especially after one of their entertainments. More disturbing, she noticed dark spots beginning to appear on her arms, along with some intermittent blurred vision. She scheduled an evaluation with her ophthalmologist, who confirmed that her vision had deteriorated just a bit, and referred her to her primary care physician about the dark spots. It was that doctor—to Marion's shock—who asked about her drinking. Blood work indicated that Marion's liver, though not in the pathological zone, did show some signs of inflammation.

Marion shared her health concerns with David, who had long been vigilant about his health. Several years before retiring, he'd had two stents surgically installed following a heart attack and had been on a blood thinner ever since. Though he was experiencing no notable symptoms other than, like Marion, some disturbed sleep and resulting lethargy, he began to wonder about his own drinking. He was aware that it had increased, but until then he had not really given it a second thought. But after his conversation with Marion, he began researching the issue of drinking and cardiac problems, and to his dismay he learned that the amount he now regularly drank did in fact put his heart health at risk.

In addition to the physical effects of alcohol, Marion and David's lifestyle had also slowly begun to hollow out in comparison to what it had been. For example, they now rarely devoted an evening to playing a board game; instead, they spent more time sitting on a couch watching television. They also went to bed somewhat earlier, despite not sleeping as well. Their walks became less frequent and shorter.

Marion and David now found themselves at a crossroads. On the one hand, they did not want to abandon the new "renovated" lifestyle they'd created; on the other hand, that same renovation appeared to pose a health risk to both of them, along with having consequences for their relationship. Not only had they renovated their living space and their social network, expanding both so as to make them more comfortable and conducive to an altered lifestyle, but it had also resulted in a significant increase in their drinking. So, what to do?

The couple decided to talk to another colleague, a retired professor in the college's counseling program. Together they went over a variety of options, ranging from abandoning the new lifestyle altogether, to cutting down on their drinking, to trying out being a sober couple. They decided on the last of these. That would be easier, Marion said, than "wasting a lot of time counting drinks."

The new lifestyle renovations that David and Marion decided on began by removing all alcohol from the house. They had a small cabinet that had been their bar, and they emptied it. Then they let their friends know that, on the advice of their doctors, they'd decided to take a break from drinking, without offering any timeline. They did not tell their friends that they could not drink at their social gatherings. Instead, they told them that moving forward, the occasions would be BYOB, or "bring your own beverage." David and Marion still held their little soirees, and occasionally another couple might bring a bottle of wine or some flavored hard seltzer. To their pleasant surprise, however, many of their friends were satisfied with appetizers, lively conversation, and mocktails.

The idea of making a lifestyle renovation, as Marion and David did, can become an issue when a couple decides to change their identity from a drinking couple to a sober couple. Such renovations often have spillover effects into various aspects of a couple's overall lifestyle. The physical and social changes Marion and David originally made after retiring (which in many ways were positive) had an unintended impact on their drinking. The same was true for Helen and Ted (discussed in chapter 4), who moved to a retirement community only to find themselves slowly caught in a web of excessive drinking, ostensibly in the context of enjoying their retirement.

Before moving on, let's pause for a moment and consider the following questions. Better still, have a discussion about them:

- Have there been any significant changes in your lifestyle as a couple in the past few years? If so, can you connect the changes in your drinking habits to these changes in your lives?
- Have you made any significant modifications to your living conditions in the past few years? Again, have any of these "renovations" coincided with changes in drinking habits?
- Can you identify any shared pleasures that have fallen by the wayside as a consequence of drinking?

ACCOMMODATION

David and Marion and Helen and Ted are good examples of how purposefully changing a lifestyle can result in an increase in drinking. The same thing can happen when one partner in a couple takes a new job that involves a lot of socializing (and drinking) or when a couple finds themselves in a new, drinking culture. The reverse is also true, however, that the changes in drinking that occur as a couple gradually slips along the drinking spectrum can also affect a couple's lifestyle. In a word, their lifestyle gradually comes to *accommodate* their drinking.

MATT AND ANIKA

Matt and Anika were an example of such accommodation. They both had jobs at a social media company in a highly competitive industry. Staying ahead of the competition in social media often means fiscal life or death corporations. It also typically means long working hours, either at the office or remotely. Matt, with a background in computer science and software design, worked in product development, while Anika worked in the marketing division. The company had successfully passed the start-up phase, where innovation along with almost compulsive hard work had paid off, but where continued prosperity depended on ongoing comparable effort and results. For many employees at their level of expertise, that meant long hours and seemingly interminable meetings analyzing concepts for new products for their feasibility and profitability or modifying existing products to increase sales.

The company was organized into teams that worked together on various aspects of product design, development, and testing. This arrangement made not only for increased productivity (several heads being better than one when it came to complex tasks), but also supported a serious work ethic. Virtually all employees had laptops that they transported between home and office, allowing work to continue unabated across what once had been a useful boundary. And it typically did just that, meaning that employees' personal lives now needed to accommodate work. That was certainly true for Matt and Anika, who often found themselves putting in time on their laptops after dinner during the week as well as on the weekends.

Neither Matt nor Anika, who met in college and dated for three years before marrying, had been much of a drinker. Both began their drinking careers not long after getting their jobs in the high-pressure world of the Internet. It turned out this was easy to do, since the team concept was conducive not only to office work but also to socializing. Friday happy hours were common, as were business-related gatherings (such as those celebrating new contracts) that included complementary wine and beer along with food. Matt and Anika fell into this social network by virtue of the fact that it was so readily available and popular. Over time, their environment began to affect their drinking. But the opposite also proved to be true: drinking changed their lifestyle in a negative, synergistic way.

Although this drinking culture was valued as a sort of built-in social network, there was a corporate policy about excessive drinking. But there was also an unwritten acknowledgment that some people overdid it. It was an open secret that some employees actually brought liquor to work (most often wine or spiked seltzer), usually in water bottles. Apparently, this was also tacitly tolerated as long as the employee performed at the expected high-functioning level, which meant working between 50 and 60 hours a week between home and office. It was assumed that the alcohol was used to help cope with stress—to "chill out" so one could work harder.

Matt and Anika began drinking more in the context of the built-in drinking culture at work, but in time they also drank more at home after work. They started with trendy low-alcohol drinks like hard cider and flavored spiked seltzer. Slowly they found a preference for wine, especially Chardonnay, which they liked to keep cold.

Over the course of about a year, Anika and Matt's lifestyle changed to accommodate the increased role that drinking had come to play in their lifestyle, including the following:

- They purchased a special wine refrigerator lined with racks for storing wine bottles, keeping their wine chilled at what was advertised as an ideal temperature.
- They purchased a couch that featured side-by-side reclining chairs as well as cupholders.
- They purchased stemless wine glasses that could fit in the cupholders.
- They'd started buying wine by the case, instead of by the bottle.

In every one of the above instances, we could make the case that it was not some change in their lifestyle that led to more drinking, but that more drinking itself had led to changes in lifestyle. In other words, their lifestyle changed to *accommodate* more drinking.

It didn't stop there. Matt then decided that he wanted to try mixing some vodka with juices, like orange juice or cranberry juice, to imitate the spiked drinks they'd come to like, but at a more potent level. He did not take the time to reflect on the fact that his own father had had a significant drinking problem—one that had cost him two jobs as well as diagnoses of hypertension and diabetes. Anika had no such history, but instead of vodka and juice, she just stuck with two (and sometimes three) glasses of Chardonnay and maybe two cans of spiked seltzer a night, starting while preparing dinner and ending at bedtime. Noticeably, their sex life had dwindled slowly over this time, though neither one of them had yet complained about it.

In time, Matt and Anika altered their daily routine in other ways to accommodate both work and drinking. For example, in order to be able to satisfy the unwritten expectation of putting in at least 50 hours a week, they took to firing up their laptops as soon as they got home from the office, working another hour or so each night. During this time they would have at least one drink. Only then would they prepare some dinner and get ready to "relax," which meant sitting on their couch with cupholders (with wine or vodka) and watching the news. Eventually they also purchased two tables where they could place their dinners while watching television and drinking.

Despite their slipping at least into the middle of the mild zone on the drinking spectrum (with Matt perhaps being at the moderate level), neither Matt nor Anika believed that they had a drinking problem because they did not get drunk, which they equated with passing out. The main consequence associated with their drinking lifestyle up to that point was a gradual loss of stamina, but they attributed it to their demanding jobs rather than drinking. But then another issue came up.

After two years of success at work, Matt's and Anika's salaries plus bonuses had increased to the point where they began to consider buying their own condominium. Anika wanted a condo with three bedrooms: one for them, one as a shared office, and one for a baby. While Matt was on board with the idea of starting a family, he also reacted with some anxiety. Specifically, he raised the issue of work and finances. Would Anika be able to continue at her job (and at the same pace) if they had a child? Would Matt be able to make up any shortfall? How much would they be paying for childcare? The issue of how their drinking lifestyle would accommodate parenthood, though, didn't come up.

Anika recognized Matt's concerns, but she stuck to her desire to have a family and not just a marriage. A few of their friends seemed to be happy being childless, but that idea held little appeal for Anika. In the end, she and Matt agreed to look to buy a condo. Meanwhile, they would begin trying to get pregnant.

Soon they faced a challenge on the pregnancy front, and it had to do with Anika's menstrual cycle. While once as consistent as clockwork, it had become increasingly irregular over the past couple of years. Though she'd avoided worrying about it until then, their plan to have a baby motivated her to consult her obstetrician. That was when the issue of drinking came up, in the form of her responses to a few questions on an inventory that Anika was asked to take before her next appointment. On reading through her answers, Anika's obstetrician told her that it was possible that drinking—especially as much as Anika admitted to—could be the culprit behind her erratic cycle. That came as a shock to Anika. She shared her desire to look to getting pregnant in the not-so-distant future. "Well," the doctor replied, "I can tell you that an occasional drink does not seem to have any significant effect on a woman's cycle, but the amount you say you drink most definitely can. It would also be a definite risk to any pregnancy."

On bringing this news home, Anika told Matt that she had already made a decision to stop drinking. Her declaration put Matt on the spot, for a couple of reasons. First, he had to face the prospect of not drinking in a show of support for Anika. Second, as it turned out, his own drinking was somewhat further along on the drinking spectrum than Anika's. For example, he'd started to surreptitiously bring some hard seltzer to work in his water bottle. He was also the one who'd been drinking vodka along with wine pretty much every night. Again, while not falling down drunk, he was definitely intoxicated on a regular basis. He realized that it would likely be a challenge for him to give up this habit, much more so than Anika, and he said so. Anika sympathized with his concerns but suggested that it would be a lot easier for her if they both decided to quit.

The couple decided that their best course, given the overall situation, was to consult with a therapist, one with expertise in counseling around the issue of drinking. Anika's doctor recommended two such counselors. The plan they came up with was that both Matt and Anika would quit drinking, at least for the foreseeable future. To make that goal easier to achieve, they would reduce the time they spent socializing, particularly the work-related kind, like happy hours, that always involved drinking. Anika volunteered that she would offer a simple explanation—something like "I've been having some stomach problems, so I'm not drinking until it gets resolved"— which she found prompted some sympathy and good wishes, but no skepticism. Matt, in contrast, had a reputation for liking his drinks, often ordering the "martini of the day" that many bars promoted, and after that he'd always drink more after returning home.

Despite the best of intentions, Matt was not able to keep up his part of their commitment. Though he truly loved Anika as well as their relationship, after three weeks he'd already drank twice with work colleagues and then again at home. Though he was still not drinking to the point of drunkenness, it was always obvious to Anika when he'd been drinking. She kept to her own commitment to be sober but pressed the issue of Matt's drinking. She was beginning to worry, she said, that Matt might prove to be a father whose drinking compromised his ability to be an effective, involved parent. That comment hit Matt hard, so much so that he brought it up at their next counseling session. He did not, he said, have any intention of becoming an "absentee father," which was how he described his own father, who also had a long-standing habit of drinking after work and then retiring early. His father was never abusive, Matt said, but neither was he very present in Matt's life. "He was not the kind of dad that a son could rely on," Matt explained.

For Matt, sober love eventually meant reaching out for additional support. He found that in part through the fellowship of SMART Recovery. He started out by listening in on some online meetings. His initial expectation, he said, was that the people in the meetings would turn out to be "losers"—men and women whose lives had been devastated by drinking or drugs. But that wasn't true at all. Many of the participants were like him: having decided to pursue sobriety but needing social support to do so. Like him, the social networks they circulated in promoted at least some amount of drinking and considered that "normal," whereas sobriety was somehow "abnormal." Unfortunately, these social networks included friends, family, and even colleagues. In his SMART meetings, however, Matt found men and women who shared a common goal. They did not judge but simply relied on one another to stay sober, often in the face of challenges.

Six months later, Matt was sober, and he and Anika were well into the process of looking at condominiums. While they both initially expressed concerns about keeping up with their work commitments (and income) should Anika become pregnant, she reported that she was experiencing significantly more energy since becoming sober and was not concerned about being able to keep pace. She did add, though, that given her skill set and experience, she was prepared to look for alternative employment in the event that proved necessary. She was confident she could succeed at that.

CLOSING THE LOOP

Participating in online (and later in-person) SMART meetings helped Matt stay sober. He was able to share his difficulties, such as the physical urges to drink that sometimes washed over him. He accepted advice from his peers about how they dealt with these urges and made steady progress, for example, by altering their routines on arriving home after work, even changing the "relaxing" clothing they'd come to associate with drinking. Still, two months into his commitment, Matt found himself succumbing to urges on two occasions. His typical slip involved stopping into a favored liquor store after work and buying two vodka "nips," which he'd consume before arriving at home. Anika was able to tell that he'd been drinking, both by the way he looked and the smell of vodka on his breath. She did not castigate him, but she did suggest they should talk to their counselor about it.

At that point Matt consulted a physician who was experienced in helping patients quit drinking. The doctor praised Matt for his progress and prescribed two medications: one that helped reduce anxiety but was also used to help promote sobriety, and one that tended to block drinking urges while reducing any alcohol high from consumed drinks. That, plus SMART Recovery, did the trick for Matt.

The final step that Anika and Matt took to support their new identity as a sober couple involved renovating their lifestyle on the physical level. The incentive for that came when Anika mentioned realizing how much they had come to alter the physical layout of their home as their drinking had progressed—how their lifestyle had come to accommodate drinking. She labeled their altered family room with its couch, cupholders, and tables facing their large television as "our drinking room." She insisted on trading that setting with a new couch with no cupholders, then got Matt to agree to having meals at the table they'd bought shortly after getting married, which was located in the kitchen next to the family room. That meant that they would also be able to communicate more over meals, instead of silently watching television as they ate (and drank).

There were additional changes. One important one was that Matt ceased bringing his spiked "water bottle" to work. Instead, he didn't bring any water bottle at all, but rather bought one or two every day at the company cafeteria. By this time they had no alcohol in their home, and they decided together to make some other changes in their routine. One of these was to take up an old, lost shared pleasure from the early days of their relationship: watching nature and history shows. They especially liked ones that depicted faraway places and political dramas. They also invested in some decent hiking shoes and poles and took to hiking together (another former shared pleasure) on weekends. Finally, they devoted considerable time scouting out areas where they might want to live and raise a family, including schools and community resources. At that point they were both invested in sober love and on the way to being very happy as a sober couple.

MOVING FORWARD

The couples described here illustrate a couple of issues that readers of this book may face. First, they illustrate how drinking, as it progresses from low risk into at least the mild and perhaps the moderate zones on the drinking spectrum, has the effect of hollowing out or eroding relationships. As time passes, the bonds that initially connected a couple tend to wither. In that sense, "recovery" for couples means reversing the hollowing-out process, which may mean resurrecting and recovering those things that helped create the bond between them in the first place. This includes things like common values and shared goals, as well as shared intimacy.

In addition to the hollowing-out process associated with progressive drinking, relationships are vulnerable to changing as drinking progresses. A couple may deliberately renovate their lifestyle—often as part of a life transition—in a way that unintentionally promotes more drinking, as happened for the newly retired David and Marion. But this accommodation can also work in the opposite direction: an increase in drinking can shape the couple's lifestyle, as happened to Matt and Anika. As you and your partner work toward sober love, it may be worthwhile to contemplate the following:

- Has any progression along the drinking spectrum led to lifestyle changes that *accommodate* drinking? What sort of changes have there been?
- Have these lifestyle changes led to you sacrificing previously pleasurable activities in favor of drinking?
- What if any of these accommodations can you reverse in the interest of becoming a sober couple?

Questions like these can spur a dialogue between you, hopefully providing a blueprint for change.

Chapter 10

REKINDLING INTIMACY

FEW OF MY CLIENTS would deny that physical, sexual attraction played a significant role at the start of their relationship. It may not be the sole factor that drew them to one another. Compatibility (shared interests, shared values, and a shared sense of humor, for example) are additional factors that couples frequently mention when they are asked about what first attracted them to their partners. In short, courting couples typically just feel comfortable together, and they are motivated by that comfortability to stay close. The British writer Marie Stopes put it succinctly when she wrote in 1918, "Every heart desires a mate."

While the above may be true for most of us, we must recognize that there are men and women today who feel no such need for a partner. Individuals who are perfectly happy on their own are not the intended audience for this book. Those who do want a life partner, though, *are* inclined to desire intimacy, including sexual intimacy. Stopes, writing in her book *Married Love*, put it this way when describing physical intimacy: "From whom there should be no concealment, whose body should be as dear to one, in every part, as one's own, and with whom all openness of interchange should establish itself."

Stopes, as an early advocate for birth control at a time when Victorian sexual repression was beginning to wane, helped to open the door for couples to talk openly about sex, including enjoying it and understanding how it contributed to their shared bond. As flowery as her language might be, many couples attest that they relate to the idea of love that Stopes puts words to. Her concept of married love was not at all pornographic; rather, it was *intimate*. Today, despite living in what we might call a pornographic culture, many couples still yearn for an intimate sexual relationship.

But the fact of the matter is that as drinking goes, so goes intimacy—and very often sex—for couples who progress along the drinking spectrum. There is progressively less intimate talk, fewer intimate activities, less affection, and less sex. That is part of the hollowing out that is a consequence of drinking as it moves away from the low-risk zone and into the mild and moderate zones and the "relationship" with drinking gets stronger. Those who desire sober love, choosing to change their identity and become a sober couple, stand to recover that lost intimacy.

HANNAH AND BEN

We've seen with other couples how drinking can progressively erode a sex life, but let's take a moment to look a bit more closely at this process. Hannah and Ben first met in high school and dated steadily for a year. They said they were both attracted to one another on a physical level. He was, she said, "tall, dark, and handsome, and not a show-off like some of the other boys." In Ben's eyes, Hannah was simply "a blond goddess." They waited to have sex until their senior year, at Hannah's insistence, though they certainly engaged in everything short of that before then—and often.

After graduating high school, Ben and Hannah elected, despite their continued attraction, to attend different colleges in different states. She left for the Ivy League, where she majored in art, while Ben opted for a highly ranked state university where he first studied business but later switched to pre-law. Despite the separation, they maintained contact, mostly over school vacations, and found that their mutual attraction did not lose its power.

After graduating, Hannah moved back to their suburban home-town and found a position as the administrative assistant to the di-rector of an art museum located in a nearby city. Ben took the Law School Admission Test (LSAT), scored well, and was accepted into the law school at the same university he'd gone to as an undergrad-uate. His parents paid for his degree, so he attended full-time, fin-ished in three years, and passed the bar exam on his first try.

Through all the undergraduate years and Ben's law school years, their sex life continued to be vibrant. Their mutual attraction was unabated, though it sometimes could be somewhat infrequent on account of Ben's academic demands. After Ben passed the bar exam, though, they had more time together, including more inti-macy. They got engaged, and both families were overjoyed.

For their first two years of marriage, Ben worked in a large law firm. The salary was good, but he did not enjoy the work environment, particularly the intense pressure to produce "billable hours." With Hannah's support (along with some modest financial backing from his parents), Ben struck out on his own and opened the independent practice he would have for the extended future. At first, Hannah worked with him part time, serving as a kind of unpaid paralegal, organizing files and helping Ben prepare for the next day's appoint-ments. Her contributions to the success of the practice were such that in a short time they'd managed to save enough to put a down pay-ment on their first house. Success continued unabated after that.

At the time they sought counseling, Hannah and Ben had been married for 17 years and had a 15-year-old son who attended a private boarding school, where he was an A student as well as an outstanding soccer player. Ben's law practice was quite successful. It was also busy, and he now employed one full-time and one part-time paralegal, plus a full-time administrative assistant. Hannah, meanwhile, had moved on from the art world and was now an editor at a successful publishing house. Finances were no issue for them, and they enjoyed life in an upscale suburban community. The issue that eventually complicated this lifestyle, however, proved to be about drinking.

The reasons why drinking turned out to be a problem for Hannah and Ben had a lot to do with how their lifestyle as a couple had gradually changed over time. In a word, it had gradually promoted more drinking, and drinking more in turn had led them to *accommodate* it in many ways. These changes were driven initially by the social life they had migrated into. That included frequent business-related social events, some involving attorneys' associations and others real estate and local business groups that wanted to cultivate business with one another as well as with Ben. Then there were family events, which also invariably included drinking. Of these, however, the business events were the boozier affairs. Hannah and Ben did have friends there and looked forward to these occasions. It was well known that drinking was a central part of this social network—and even that some people were prone to overindulging—but it continued to thrive nevertheless.

Their gradual immersion in this drinking culture, combined with their son being away most of the time, led the couple to extend their drinking to their time at home, where Ben looked forward to his nightly single malt scotch on the rocks, and Hannah enjoyed vodka and tonic. In time, their consumption gradually increased to the point where Ben increasingly fell asleep while watching television in a lounge chair (which he'd insisted on buying so he could relax while having his drinks), only coming to bed when he awoke around three o'clock in the morning.

It was Hannah who first broached the issue of drinking, at one point suggesting that it was playing a major role in what she labeled a "deterioration" of their marriage. She even went so far one night as to accuse Ben of getting drunk every night, to which he took great offense. And while she acknowledged her own drinking had increased, Hannah insisted it fell well short of Ben's.

This schism in their relationship eventually led to arguments, with Hannah saying that their marriage was falling apart and Ben defensively arguing that Hannah was exaggerating things. He added that if he was guilty of falling asleep on the lounge chair, she was guilty of falling asleep in bed while posting on social media. In the end, Hannah got Ben to agree to see a counselor with her.

Asked by the counselor at their first visit to describe their current lifestyle, they explained that their "shared pleasures" currently consisted mainly of eating in nice restaurants two or three times a week and attending a business-related social event once a week. These meals, while appealing, tended to be highly caloric. There was also a lot of alcohol. They had gained weight, especially Ben, who was put on a low dose of hypertensive medication by his doctor, who encouraged some dieting and weight loss. For her part, Hannah had also put on some weight, and her own doctor suggested this contributed to the swelling she sometimes experienced in her knees. "Lose a few pounds," he advised, "and the swelling will probably go down."

Although in the past they had taken regular walks in a nearby park, Ben and Hannah couldn't recall the last time they went on one. They had a swimming pool but rarely used it. They'd also once enjoyed the theatre but hadn't attended a show in two years. They had a dog, Max, whom Ben used to regularly walk on weekdays in their neighborhood. Now, however, Max's exercise consisted mainly of running around in a small fenced-in area in their backyard. These days their usual daily routine—other than a meal out or a social event—involved retreating to separate rooms at home, where Ben would watch television while sipping his scotch on the rocks while Hannah occupied herself on her tablet.

Asked about intimacy between them, Hannah was to one to speak out, and rather forcefully at that, for it seemed that sex had become an increasingly rare occurrence between them. And even when they did have sex, Ben was often unable to keep an erection long enough to complete intercourse.

While Ben blushed at this interchange, the counselor calmly pointed out that both Ben and Hannah seemed to drink a lot more than what could be considered a "social" or "low-risk" level, and that drinking as much as they did most likely contributed to Ben's sexual dysfunction. The counselor added that it could affect Hannah's sexual performance too, as alcohol tends to reduce testosterone, the hormone that plays a role in libido. Reduced testosterone levels as a result of heavy drinking, he explained, could account for their lack of sexual interest.

This news left the couple in a quandary. The counselor asked them to put aside some time over the next two weeks to sit together and take stock of how their lifestyle had changed over the past several years, and specifically how drinking had come to play a more central role in their lives. How did their shared pleasures today, including physical intimacy of any kind, compare to when they first married? What other shared pleasures may have declined? Would they be interested in recovering any of those shared pleasures? Would they be interested in rekindling sexual intimacy?

A BLUEPRINT FOR CHANGE

Despite the fact that they had undeniably drifted apart over time, neither Ben nor Hannah reported being so unhappy with their marriage that they would consider ending it. Rather, they both acknowledged that the changes in their relationship had happened gradually, and that they wanted to improve their relationship. While on some level they both recognized how things had changed, they hesitated to face it, in a kind of conspiracy of silence. Moreover, they recognized that the hollowing out of their relationship was correlated with gradual changes in their drinking habits, changes that were influenced by their overall lifestyle. This new lifestyle, particularly at home, had in turn changed so as to accommodate drinking. Ben then asked a common question: "So what do we do, abandon the social life and relationships we've developed over the past two decades?"

While Ben's question acknowledged the formidable challenge at hand, the first thing he and Hannah needed to do was decide if they wanted to continue down the path they were on, or consider making a radical change in their relationship. In other words, they needed to decide if they were going to become a sober couple. Fortunately, their love for one another, combined with their shared devotion to their relationship and their son (who they agreed they did not want to see becoming a heavy drinker) proved enough for them to undertake a truly radical change in their lifestyle.

RENOVATIONS

Although Hannah and Ben agreed to the new goal of becoming a sober couple, they worried about how they were going to achieve it. They were intelligent people, and it was obvious to them that simply trying to not drink might very well be a path to failure without also

making other significant changes. Their counselor agreed, and together they developed a blueprint for pursuing shared sobriety that
would prove to be robust and resilient over time. That blueprint re-
volved around a plan to renovate their lifestyle. It was ambitious, but
together with their counselor, they decided to work on it a piece at a
time, without alcohol. Here are some elements of the plan that Hannah and Ben devised:

- *Substituting nonalcoholic beverages for alcohol.* Ben and Hannah told friends, family, and business associates that they had
  decided to forego drinking for health reasons (shared weight
  and mobility problems, Ben's hypertension). At the same time,
  they began skipping some business-related social activities in
  favor of staying home, enjoying a low-calorie dinner together,
  and taking a walk. They also decided to limit any drinking to
  nonalcoholic beverages.
- *Removing alcohol from their home.* This proved to be more difficult than they expected. Hannah admitted that she missed
  her nightly drinks once the vodka was gone. But it was Ben
  who was really suffering. He admitted to feeling frustrated
  that he could not have his beloved single malt scotch. After two
  weeks of sobriety, Ben stated in counseling that he was experiencing regular cravings to drink, had dreamed about drinking, and had even thought more than once of taking his car for
  a "scotch run" to his favorite liquor store. With the support of
  their counselor, however, they did "bite the bullet" and dis-
  posed of the contents of their liquor cabinet.
- *Trying a recovery fellowship.* In further discussions with their
  counselor, and given Ben's inner struggles, the idea of reaching out to a recovery fellowship like AA was raised. Ben could
  admit that his drinking had progressed along the drinking

spectrum over time, yet he bristled at the idea of being diagnosed as an alcoholic. Hannah, who had decided to research
AA a bit, brought up the fact that AA's stated goal did not use
diagnoses; rather, its sole criterion for being involved was "a
desire to stop drinking." Ben said that he did satisfy that criterion. Moreover, he knew of several attorneys who were in
recovery and attended AA. He decided to reach out to two of
them, and they encouraged him to try out a couple of online
AA meetings, including one that had been started by and for
attorneys. He decided to have a talk with his doctor, too. The
doctor told Ben that he probably would qualify for a diagnosis
of alcohol dependence, for two reasons: it seemed that Ben
currently drank enough that there was always some alcohol in
his body, and he experienced an urge to drink virtually every
day. He offered to prescribe medication that could help reduce
Ben's cravings if he wanted it, though Ben decided to put that
on hold for now. He decided instead to try out a couple of the
online meetings his colleagues mentioned. Ben discovered,
somewhat to his surprise, that they were extremely helpful. He
found that just by listening, he could identify with these colleagues who described similar histories as well as current
struggles. They also made themselves available to talk through
urges when they occurred, as well as to strategize ways to stay
sober rather than give in to that urge to drink.

· *Rearranging the house.* Ben and Hannah agreed that their
nightly habit of retreating to separate rooms had to change—
physically. Again, Ben was more resistant, arguing that Hannah might complain about his choice of television programs,
which were heavily weighted toward crime and mystery series
(including a few legal dramas). But Hannah only laughed and
said that she would have no problem getting a pair of noise-

canceling headphones. She said that she would like to get back to her former pleasure—reading—especially about art and artists. The counselor then asked Hannah if she had any other suggestions, to which she responded that she would like to resume the walks they'd once enjoyed, even if they were short ones. The word "short" appealed to Ben, and he agreed. As a final touch, the counselor suggested that they replace Ben's beloved lounge chair with some new comfortable furniture and place it in the room they would now be sharing. Ben, initially skeptical, later admitted that not sitting in the lounge chair he associated with drinking was helpful. That provision seemed to satisfy the need for physical renovations, at least for now.

MOTIVATED BY SOBER LOVE

After a year of shared sobriety, Ben and Hannah, now a sober couple, told their counselor, whom they now still met with monthly, that they had no intention of returning to drinking. They'd experienced too many positive consequences of sober love to contemplate reversing course. By that time, the positives were many:

- They were both physically healthier. They'd both lost some weight (enough to facilitate more activity), Ben's doctor was able to reduce the dosage of his blood pressure medication, and Hannah had regained a significant amount of her mobility.
- Their lifestyle was no longer hollowed out. Their daily and weekly routines now included strolls through the park, swimming in their pool, and watching television series together twice a week. Ben had even come home with a jigsaw puzzle of a Scottish castle (which they now planned to visit).

- They'd spent a week vacationing in the Outer Banks with their son and enjoyed daily walks along the beach.
- Their sex life had experienced something of a renewal. They'd even experimented with a sex toy (a vibrator) that Ben had brought home. At first they'd both laughed, but after giving it a try, they gave up laughing in favor of more erotic vocalizations.
- They maintained an active (but sober) social life. They experienced no discomfort letting friends, family, and colleagues know that they were now a sober couple, and for many reasons. In fact, Hannah said that she'd been approached by a few friends asking how they'd decided and then managed to become a sober couple.

It's clear that embracing a new identity as a sober couple for Ben and Hannah involved more than a simple decision not to drink. Such commitments are almost always short-lived. Like many New Year's resolutions, they tend to be superficial, are not well thought out, and lack any detail or plan that can sustain them. Fortunately, Hannah and Ben had a long-standing, solid relationship and open, honest communication. The strength of their relationship allowed them first to take a look at their drinking and where it had led them, and then to reach out for help so as not to go it alone. That included counseling and, for Ben, taking advantage of a recovery fellowship that supported but did not judge him, where he found men and women he could identify with as he struggled to overcome both urges to drink and a lifestyle that had come to accommodate drinking.

Another factor that no doubt contributed to Ben and Hannah's success, aside from their shared commitment to their marriage, was the fact that they experienced no shame in changing the direction of their lives in favor of sobriety. This can be a challenge for many couples, given the reality of our current drinking culture. Many expect to be greeted with skepticism, or even subtle ridicule, for making such a decision. Yet Ben and Hannah's experience is more the rule than the exception. Even so, they agreed that any friends who could not accept their new identity as a couple were probably not truly friends at all.

FURTHER FOOD FOR THOUGHT
ON REKINDLING INTIMACY

As intimacy gradually fades as a consequence of a couple's drinking lifestyle, many say that the idea of recovering or "rekindling" intimacy, especially sexual intimacy, can present an awkward, even intimidating challenge. Some say that they hesitate to initiate any kind of physical contact—outside perhaps of a quick and pro-forma hug—simply because it has faded from their relationship, and they are now shy to reintroduce it. Some may have experienced sexual dysfunction, a frequent consequence of regular drinking in the moderate zone on the spectrum, and now fear failure and embarrassment. Others, meanwhile, may hesitate out of sexual anxiety. They may, for example, have had a negative sexual experience in their past that translates into anxiety when affection gets physical. This may prompt more drinking as a way of disinhibiting their sexuality. Suzanne, whom we discussed in chapter 3, came to rely on drinking to overcome shame about her sexual orientation and allow her to act on her desire. For individuals like Suzanne, I recommend involvement in one of the fellowships described here, plus ongoing psychotherapy with a counselor experienced in helping people deal with the effects of trauma.

As much as couples may hesitate to broach the issue of rekindling intimacy, they stand to gain a great deal by adding this component to being a sober couple. In doing so, the first and best rule is: *Don't rush.* Professionals who specialize in helping couples overcome a blocked sexual relationship, beginning with the ground-breaking work of Masters and Johnson in the 1970s, know that anxiety created by trying to move too fast and expecting too much too soon can lead to failure and frustration. Couples often make more progress by giving themselves the space to move at a comfortable pace toward rekindling intimacy. The hollowing-out consequences of drinking didn't happen overnight; addressing those issues won't happen overnight, either. Frank and Mary are an example of a couple who did rekindle their intimacy successfully, much to their great satisfaction.

FRANK AND MARY

Frank and Mary had been a sober couple for nearly a year, having been together for 28 years, and married for 26. Their decision to become a sober couple had been precipitated in large measure by Mary suffering a heart attack, which luckily turned out to be relatively mild and from which she had fully recovered. Yet heart problems ran in her family, and she recognized that over a decade or more her affinity for cocktails—especially sugary ones—had led to her being a daily drinker. So was Frank, who preferred beer produced in local microbreweries. They found that they were able to succeed in their goal of sobriety mostly through a shared commitment and mutual support, along with some renovations in their daily and weekend routines. When Mary explained her reasons for quitting, their two grown sons and sole daughter-in-law supported their decision wholeheartedly, as did their friends.

At this point the rack that had held Frank's beer stein collection was gone from the kitchen counter. In its place was an expensive blender they used to make fruit smoothies, along with a flavored seltzer maker. The freestanding cabinet that once held liquor and various mixers had been donated to charity.

Both Frank and Mary attested that the decision to become a sober couple was worthwhile. They both felt that they had renewed energy, had lost some weight through mild but regular exercise and an improved diet, and were more active on weekends than they had been for quite a while. But Mary did have one issue that she felt compelled to bring up, and that was the fact that they had not had sex in a long time—"longer than I can remember," she said. Frank, though embarrassed, had to agree, but he blamed himself for the decline, specifically problems he'd had keeping an erection. He added that he did miss sex, especially since it had once been a vibrant part of their relationship, but then added that he was wary, expecting to encounter the same problem if they attempted intercourse.

Mary was able to understand Frank's dilemma, but she didn't want to stop there. She also had some reservations, wondering if she would still be capable of having an orgasm after being "out of practice" for so long. Nevertheless, she went online and located a therapist who had experience with sexual dysfunction and persuaded Frank, who after all was still interested in sex, to meet with this therapist.

The therapist turned out to be a woman, whose first item of agenda was to ask Frank if he was okay talking about sex with a woman therapist, in response to which he shrugged. The therapist explained that this was a fairly common reaction but that she had helped many men and women overcome such issues. She then ascertained that neither Frank nor Mary had any medical issues that might cause a sexual dysfunction, but that their shared drinking history could well have been a culprit. She explained that her approach, which had a track record of success, was to avoid moving too quickly in restoring intimacy, which she defined as something "including sex, but also bigger than sex."

The therapist wanted to work with Frank and Mary collaboratively "to add more to the intimacy dimension" of their relationship, beginning with their relationship out of the bedroom. This idea surprised Frank, and he said so, but added that he also felt relieved. Over the next month, they developed an addition to the lifestyle renovations they had already made, one that pleased them both. First, they had a four-person hot tub installed in the three-season porch that looked out onto their backyard. This room also had a table and four comfortable chairs, none of which had seen a lot of use since their sons had moved on. Now, however, their daughter-in-law joked that they would have to visit more often!

To add to the hot tub, Frank purchased a portable fire pit for the backyard. One of his greatest pleasures growing up, he said, was to sit by the fire with his father and soak up the heat from the flames on a cool fall evening. Around the fire pit they added two lawn chairs.

Next, they made a commitment to using the hot tub at least twice a week and the fire pit whenever Frank wanted to, which turned out to be one night every weekend. Together they would sit by the fire pit while sharing tasty appetizers from a local restaurant or just some good cheese and crackers, along with flavored seltzer. After eating, they moved to the hot tub, where they soaked up the warmth and relaxed.

Their therapist then took the step of suggesting that Frank and Mary move to the bedroom after relaxing in their hot tub. She cautioned, however, that her aim was still to avoid unrealistic expectations. She therefore suggested that they purchase some pleasant massage oil and take turns giving each other a ten-minute massage in the bedroom, adding they might also consider playing some soothing instrumental music. Finally—and this was most important—they were not to put intercourse or orgasm on the agenda for now. Frank may experience a partial erection, or Mary might begin to feel aroused, but now was not the time to do anything more than enjoy those feelings along with the massage. Frank asked why.

The therapist explained that the most common cause of sexual dysfunction was something called *spectatoring*. As researchers Masters and Johnson defined it, spectatoring involves "standing outside of yourself and watching" while having sex, and all the while fearing that things will go wrong. They believed that the anxiety associated with spectatoring could in and of itself cause impaired sexual performance. Therefore an interim goal for Frank and Mary was to be able to engage in physical touch with no excessive expectations, thereby avoiding the chances of spectatoring.

As simple as it may sound, this intervention devised by Masters and Johnson often works, as it did for Frank and Mary. After a few weeks of massages twice or three nights a week, they both reported feeling sexually aroused, though they went along with the therapist's "no sex" recommendation. Then the therapist suggested they could "stimulate" one another a bit more. If Frank should get a full erection, then he and Mary could try to have intercourse, but they should not feel that he needed to continue intercourse to orgasm. It would be fine, the therapist said, if Frank could enjoy intercourse for a minute, but without expecting to go longer than that for now. She was looking for "progress, not perfection," she added. This approach also proved to be effective, and Frank said that under those circumstances he no longer "spectatored" himself, essentially standing back and wondering if he'd lose his erection.

The approach worked for Mary and Frank, and before long they were having intercourse for the first time in years, with Mary having orgasms. Frank did admit that he'd found it a bit frustrating to not pursue sex further when he first started to experience an erection, but another part of him felt relieved that the pressure was off.

For her part, Mary said she too had been enjoying the feelings of arousal, but without wondering how Frank might be doing.

Frank and Mary's story is not intended as a substitute for competent sex therapy. Rather, it's meant to illustrate how sexual intimacy can fall victim to drinking, and that it can in fact be rekindled when a couple decides to pursue sober love.

MOVING FORWARD

Recovering intimacy that is lost in a relationship as drinking takes its progressive toll is perhaps the most dramatic benefit that couples stand to experience when they elect to become sober together. Some couples say they were aware of this aspect of the hollowing out of their relationship for a long time but avoided bringing it up. In other cases, one partner would occasionally complain about a lack of intimacy, but again there would be no action taken as long as drinking continued to occupy a big slice of their relationship, and as other shared pleasures also faded.

Rekindling intimacy often strengthens a couple's motivation to embrace sober love as a central dynamic of their relationship. That being said, it's only realistic to expect a few bumps and potholes along the road to an alcohol-free lifestyle.

Chapter 11

SPIRITUALITY AND SOBER LOVE

WHEN I FIRST BEGAN to speak on the topic of spirituality, specifically the role it can play in recovery, I was greeted with a lot of skepticism. Colleagues and therapists frequently expressed opinions like these:

- "Spirituality is too vague and complex of a topic to be talked about in therapy."
- "Therapists shouldn't be telling clients what they should believe."
- "I really don't see a connection between spirituality and being sober."

Over time, I've developed two responses to such criticisms. First, I point to the growing research on spirituality and its role in choosing sobriety over drinking or drug use. Second, I like to point out that even though skeptics often equate spirituality with religion, the truth is that they are different. To be sure, virtually all religions advocate for spirituality, but one can also live a spiritual lifestyle without adhering to any formal religion.

DEFINING SPIRITUALITY

Although spirituality is often equated with religious practice, some thoughtful researchers have defined spirituality independent of religiosity. One way to think of spirituality is that it consists of the values and priorities we hold, along with how closely our day-to-day lives align with those values and priorities. That boils down in turn to the kinds of behaviors and activities we choose to engage in. This is in fact how researchers have gone about defining and studying spirituality. More about that soon.

ALCOHOL'S EFFECTS ON SPIRITUALITY

Many of the couples whose stories have been told in this book can attest to how drinking steadily deteriorated any spirituality" that may have once been present in their relationships. They will tell you that as their drinking gradually moved along the spectrum, from low risk to moderate or even severe, they increasingly acted in ways that were counter to their values and priorities, which were reflected in the lifestyle they once lived. Again, the main culprit here is how much time and energy gets devoted to drinking (how much one's lifestyle changes to accommodate alcohol) and how much other activities are gradually pushed to the wayside as a result of a growing relationship with drinking. Drinking simply absorbs more and more of the free time and energy couples once enjoyed together. Some say that drinking made them gradually more self-absorbed, leaving less time for cultivating their relationship outside of drinking.

WHAT WE KNOW ABOUT SPIRITUALITY AND SOBRIETY

Over the past decade or more, curious and creative researchers have taken on the challenge of examining how spirituality might play a role in supporting sobriety. Couples interested in a sober relationship can benefit greatly by giving some thought to these findings and how they might begin to integrate them into their new sober lifestyle.

In one study, Stephanie Carroll, a psychologist at the California School of Professional Psychology, recruited a sample of 100 members from 20 different AA groups in Northern California. Her goal was to evaluate the relationship between these men and women's spiritual practices and their sobriety. To do this, she needed first to define "spirituality" in some way, and then measure it. She chose a range of activities and measured them using a questionnaire that asked respondents how often they engaged in each of a number of activities, from daily to yearly. While these activities are not necessarily aspects of any specific religion, most would agree that they are manifestations of what we commonly think of as spirituality.

Here are some of the activities that the questionnaire asked about:

- Praying
- Meditating
- Reading spiritual material (daily affirmations or meditations)
- Spending time in nature (hiking or camping)
- Interacting with or creating art (visiting a museum, painting, or drawing)
- Listening to comforting music
- Attending a religious service
- Volunteering in community service activities or organizations

In this sample of active AA members, more than half reported praying and/or meditating twice a day as well as reading some form of spiritual literature three times a week. Half also reported listening to music that they defined as spiritual, meaning that it was music that was consistent with meditation or prayer, on a weekly basis. Half also said that they interacted with art and/or nature in some way at least monthly. Interestingly, despite these spiritual activities, less than half of the sample reported attending formal religious services.

The researcher's questionnaire also asked respondents to indicate their current length of sobriety in years and months. She then compared that to how the men and women in her sample scored on her spirituality scale. What she found was that habits such as meditation, prayer, and reading spiritual literature—as well as activities such as connecting to art or nature and community service—were significantly correlated with the length of sobriety. In other words, integrating spiritual activities into one's lifestyle was associated with a more robust recovery. Couples considering sobriety should ask themselves the following questions:

- Was there a time when you as a couple engaged in any of the activities that are consistent with Carroll's definition of spirituality?
- Did you find that any of these activities occupied less and less of your lifestyle over time?
- Are there any activities that you think would be worthwhile renewing?
- Are there new activities that you'd like to try adding to your sober lifestyle?

In a second study, a group of researchers headed by John Kelly of Harvard Medical School also examined spirituality and the role it might play in recovery. Using a large sample of 1,726 men and women who had undergone treatment for alcohol use disorders, they looked at several variables. They calculated the percentage of days abstinent (PDA) and drinks per drinking day (DDD), standard measures in substance misuse research. PDA indicates the extent to which an individual abstains totally from alcohol, while DDD measures how many drinks a person consumes on a day that they do drink.

Kelly measured spirituality by using what he called the Religious Background and Behavior (RBB) questionnaire. The RBB defines spirituality by first asking respondents to identify themselves as one of the following:

- Atheist: not believing in God.
- Agnostic: believing we can't really know about God.
- Unsure: doesn't know what to believe about God.
- Spiritual: believes in God but is not religious.
- Religious: believes in God and practices a religion.

Next, respondents to the RBB are asked to estimate how often they engage in different activities on an eight-point scale that ranges from "never" to "more than one a day." They include activities such as:

- Praying (alone or with others)
- Meditating (alone or with others)
- Attending religious services
- Reading spiritual writings
- Listening to spiritual music
- Attending spiritually related presentations or discussions (alone or with others)
- Connecting with nature

In her study of spirituality and recovery, Carroll found that the recovering men and women showed a significant correlation with spiritual beliefs, yet less than half of them attended formal religious services. Kelly and colleagues found that higher scores on spiritual activities were also positively related to PDA (abstinence) and negatively related to DDD (drinking). At the same time, fewer than half of the respondents stated that they identified themselves as religious. In other words, men and women who reported more involvement in spiritual activities were indeed more likely to remain abstinent, and to drink less if they did slip. Here again, however, only a minority reported attending formal religious services regularly.

Although some researchers claim that spirituality is too vague a concept to quantify and study scientifically, we can draw several conclusions from the above research. The first is that there is indeed a positive relationship between spirituality and sobriety. Second, incorporating some spiritual activities into their lifestyle can help a couple pursue sober love. Third, recovery-oriented fellowships such as AA, Women for Sobriety, and others whose programs advocate for spiritual values such as altruism, humility, and faith in the collective power of fellowship can also promote spiritual development.

WHAT IS A SPIRITUAL LIFE?

Another way to look at spirituality is to think of it in terms of the values and priorities we hold dear, and the degree to which we live by those values and priorities on a day-to-day basis. While it's probably safe to say that few if any of us could boast that our values and lifestyles are totally congruent, the truth is that dependence on alcohol or other substances exerts a progressively negative effect on this spiritual domain of life. As substance use progresses along the spectrum—from mild to moderate to potentially severe—men and women attest that they also progressively violate those values and priorities they once tried to live by. They may neglect commitments, abuse or exploit relationships, lie, or otherwise act in ways that would once have made them cringe. All of the fellowships discussed in this book recognize this reality and view recovery as a process of rebuilding a lifestyle consistent with one's core values.

In assessing the role of spirituality in sober love, it may be helpful for couples to think about how important each of the following values has been to them, and which may need corrective action:

- *Honesty*: The willingness to admit how you may not have lived according to your values, or faced the truth about how drinking has affected your relationship, as opposed to minimizing or denying those effects.
- *Altruism*: The capacity for empathy combined with a willingness (at least at times and when it would not do us harm) to put others' needs and welfare above our own desires.
- *Humility*: Being able to own up to your limitations as well as your strengths.

Men and women in recovery have long acknowledged how addiction hollowed out their lifestyles when it came to spirituality as defined above. As a couple pursuing sober love, it may be helpful to start a dialogue about how you might, over time, begin to recover this aspect of spirituality in your relationship.

MOVING TOWARD A MORE SPIRITUAL LIFESTYLE

The research studies reviewed here started with definitions of what it means to be spiritual and how spirituality relates to staying sober. That's about as good a guideline as we could hope for. We know from this research that spiritual practices support recovery, and also that those in recovery are inclined to increase these activities over time. Couples reading this book should keep in mind that spirituality, as defined and studied by these researchers, is not the same as religiosity. That said, couples can consider gradually adding one or more of the following to their shared lifestyle:

- *Meditation or prayer.* A good way to start each day is with a meditation. Many books, websites, and smartphone apps offer inspiring daily quotes and affirmations. Some have religious themes, others do not. Either way, meditations can help to ground you at the start of each day. Many couples I've worked with read a meditation together and then discuss it at least briefly over breakfast, coffee, or tea.
- *Community service.* Altruism is an important spiritual value, and a decision to participate in some form of community service, no matter how minor, can make a big difference in one's life. Again, most community organizations welcome couples committing whatever time they can to their activities, be that volunteering at a soup kitchen, donating to a community pantry, or making periodic home visits for our growing elderly population.
- *Connecting with art or nature.* This means spending time getting in touch with the earth that sustains us all. Join a club that sponsors nature walks (or just get outside as a couple). Visit an art museum now and then, and spend some time contemplating and talking about what you see.
- *Listen to music that soothes you.* Playing pleasant music in the company of a loved one can help promote bonding.

At its essence, spirituality is getting in touch with those values and priorities we value and would like to live by. Integrating activities consistent with these values and priorities can strengthen the kind of shared recovery we have been talking about in this book.

Chapter 12

COLORING OUTSIDE THE LINES

Love and Creativity

WHEN MY YOUNGER DAUGHTER Maggie was 7, my wife and I took her out of the public school she was in and placed her in a private Quaker school. We were not Quakers, but the school had its appeal, being located close by on a farm-like campus with lots of mature trees, a modest meeting house, and a sense of serenity. The main reason, though, was that Maggie was struggling to fit into the regular public school setting. Even at that young age, it was obvious that she possessed some unique talents that didn't make for a good fit.

In art class, the students would be asked to color line drawings of flowers, animals, and so on. But they were instructed to "color between the lines," which Maggie seemed to have trouble doing. Instead, she was inclined to color many images outside the lines. Our initial response to this was to encourage our daughter to follow the teacher's directions. This proved to be of no avail, as Maggie continued to produce colorful pictures that were often outside the lines. Things deteriorated to the point where several students started ridiculing Maggie. That's when we decided to look around for an alternative and found the Quaker school, which was fortunately affordable with our modest financial resources. After meeting with the principal and a teacher, we discovered that they found this story humorous, and they reassured us that it was okay with them if Maggie colored outside the lines.

To those who may be wondering about the point of this story, here is the ending: Maggie Nowinski (www.maggienowinski.org) is now an art professor who has had exhibitions—of paintings, watercolors, and installations—in galleries, colleges, and universities throughout New England.

COLORING OUTSIDE THE LINES AND SHARED SOBRIETY

In many ways, deciding to swim against the current and pursue sobriety as a couple in a drinking culture is much like deciding to color outside the lines. Within the fellowship of AA, for example, newly sober men and women are cautioned to avoid "emotional entanglements"—in other words, getting into a serious relationship—until they have achieved at least a year of sobriety. But what about those who are reading this book, couples who are *already* in a relationship?

GAIL AND LILA

Gail and Lila were in their late thirties and married for four years, having been a couple for five years before that. Gail was a high school special education teacher, while Lila worked as a senior editor for a combination print and online magazine. This was Gail's tenth year in the job, and she found it getting more stressful by the year. She loved her students; however, school budgets were being cut year after year, which meant that each term, additional students were assigned to her class while the paraprofessional staff that assisted her was steadily cut back. Her students included some with autism, others with significant learning disorders, plus others who had severe emotional and behavioral problems. She described herself as "super busy" during the week. Her sources of relief in the past had mainly occurred during weekends, school vacations, and summers, which she chose to take off rather than accept a summer position. Currently, though, she found herself having to devote a couple of hours a day after school preparing lessons for a diverse class the next day. She described this routine as taxing but bearable.

Gail's job was by no means easy, but Lila's job, in contrast, was something else. When she'd first begun working in this field it was at a small magazine, a strictly print product that was sold mostly through bookstores and by subscription. She described the work at that time as demanding but rewarding in terms of the final product. A big part of her job involved determining the themes for upcoming issues, hiring contract writers to produce appropriate materials, and working with the production staff and writers to put together the final product. At that time Lila was truly a low-risk drinker, consuming perhaps as many as five or six glasses of wine or one or two cocktails a week, mostly in a social context, including with Gail on weekends.

Looking back, as busy as she was at that first job, Lila described working at her current magazine—a much larger, more successful, and diversified publication that included both print and online editions—as nothing less than grueling. These days, it seemed, she was never able to really stop working. At first, the pandemic-driven decision by corporate that staff would work remotely seemed a blessed relief—until Lila discovered that this also meant that there were no longer any boundaries separating her work life from her home life. Whereas Gail would arrive home at around 3:30 each afternoon, then spend another hour or so preparing for the next day's lessons, Lila's work-related emails and texts never seemed to end. Her boss, second in command to the publisher, made it clear on a number of occasions that she expected responses from Lila, even to emails or texts sent after 10:00 p.m.

Over time, both Lila and Gail became frustrated with the demands of Lila's job. The reality was that the print business, for both magazines and newspapers, was in a state of long decline. That created a situation where if a person like Lila wanted to keep her job (which paid her fairly well), the only option was to work hard to produce a product that drew the attention of existing and potential readers, month after month. Coming up with attractive and timely themes, and then following through to publish articles that spoke to those themes in an entertaining manner, was an ongoing challenge (and stressful) to say the least. In addition, the lack of boundaries meant that the couple had less time to spend together: talking, taking walks, cooking, making love, and more. Given that reality, Lila and Gail spent what little free time they had expressing their frustrations, but also thinking and talking about options.

A significant part of Lila's job involved interacting both internally with the magazine staff to plan for future editions, and externally with the writers she contracted with to take on the job of researching and writing articles for the magazine's monthly theme. She also needed to communicate with the writers to give feedback on their first drafts. Needless to say, all of her duties, not to mention the need to keep an eye on deadlines, required a lot of time and energy.

As the COVID pandemic began to subside, Lila decided to start reporting to the office two days a week, in part to reestablish some kind of boundary between home and work. That didn't pan out too well, as the expectation to respond to texts and emails at all hours appeared to have hardened. Then Lila developed a habit of meeting writers for lunch, both to go over their assignments and to escape work for a while. Those lunches typically involved, at first, a glass of wine, but later two. Then, after work, Lila found that pouring another glass of wine helped her to unwind. This was understandable given the constant pressure she was under to produce work that was the lifeblood of the magazine. Over time, though, one glass of wine led to two, three, or more. Eventually she got into the habit of having a final glass of wine before bed. But despite being able to fall asleep quickly, she would often wake up in the middle of the night and not be able to get back to sleep.

Before meeting Lila, Gail had long been a low-risk, occasional drinker. She had a low tolerance for alcohol, and usually one glass of wine was enough to give her a "glow," as she put it. Over time, however, and as Lila's drinking slowly but steadily increased, from one to three or more glasses of wine daily, so did Gail's. Even then, two glasses of wine were more than enough to make Gail feel intoxicated. And while increased drinking sometimes led Lila to slur her words, for Gail it meant falling asleep early, often on the couch, and waking up feeling groggy.

A moment of crisis—a bump in the road—hit this couple late one evening when Lila took a call from the assistant publisher. Lila generally preferred to communicate via texts at that hour, but this time when she answered, her slurred speech must have become obvious. Her boss commented on it, then asked if Lila felt she was up to doing the editing on a feature piece they were planning on publishing in the next issue.

Lila was embarrassed by this experience. She tried covering up the next day by saying that she wasn't feeling well and had taken two over-the-counter sleep aids, which probably accounted for her speech. The assistant publisher grunted a reply, then said she had to go, leaving off that she hoped Lila would report the next day with the expected editing.

This incident led to more talk between Lila and Gail. Gail was assertive in stating that it was obvious to her—if not to Lila as yet—that Lila's alcohol consumption had increased significantly over the past couple of years. Gail acknowledged that her own drinking had increased some as well. But Gail thought that Lila truly had a "drinking problem," in that she drank every night, as well as at work lunches, and she rarely had just one glass of wine. She then suggested that Lila think about cutting down on her drinking.

Although she found this confrontation as uncomfortable as her interaction over the phone with her boss, Lila had to admit that Gail was right. She promised to cut down on her drinking. Her commitment, though, proved to be half-hearted. For the next two weeks, Lila drank every night but limited herself to two glasses of wine. But even this amount she found difficult to maintain, and within a month her drinking slowly increased back to where she'd started.

Again Gail spoke up. During this time, she had been able to cut back on her own drinking to the point where she was back in the low-risk zone on the drinking spectrum—not drinking daily and consuming fewer than six glasses of wine a week. Having reflected on their situation, she felt that the underlying problem was Lila's job, which was "driving her into the ground." Whereas she once enjoyed being an editor, it was clear to Gail at least that Lila now all but dreaded it. Moreover, their relationship was suffering because of her job. Time together was rationed. Favored activities they'd once looked forward to—golf, racquetball, attending concerts—had all fallen by the wayside. And from Gail's point of view, it was Lila's crushing workload that was to blame. She didn't believe that Lila's drinking would have become such a problem if it weren't for her job. Worst of all from Gail's perspective was that Lila had given up on what she saw as Lila's one true passion: not editing, but baking.

Lila had been raised in a small town in Upstate New York, one small enough to have been passed over by the big box retailers, but big enough to host a downtown area with a few locally owned restaurants and shops. One of these shops was a bakery owned by Lila's grandmother. It was there that Lila, beginning as a small girl, had learned the art of baking. Her mother still worked in the bakery every day. The bakery was successful, selling breads, pastries, cookies, cakes, and muffins to a committed customer base. Together, her mother and grandmother, along with a couple of hired staff, operated the bakery between the hours of 6:00 in the morning and 3:00 in the afternoon. After her grandmother "retired" (she continued to work in the bakery part time), Lila's mother took over. By adding another baker and keeping it within limits (no dining in, for example), she was able to keep the bakery open through the pandemic, even increasing its business somewhat between the combination of patrons being starved for locally baked fresh goods and wanting curbside pickup. Lila hadn't worked in the bakery since she left for college, though she took the skills she'd learned there with her and became a bit of a baking celebrity within their social circle.

Lila's response to Gail this time was that she was willing to see a counselor together to see if they could find a way to cut down on her drinking. To Lila's dismay, after spending an hour doing an assessment, the counselor offered the opinion that, given Lila's drinking habits, she didn't believe that moderation was a reasonable goal. Instead, she recommended that both Gail and Lila abstain from drinking for the next six months. She also added, catching Lila by surprise, that Lila should give some serious thought to changing jobs.

In addition to counseling and making some renovations at home (no alcohol, eating only at the kitchen table instead of in front of the television, drink in hand), Lila found that she needed support. So she joined a fellowship—Women for Sobriety—to help maintain her sobriety. But she admitted that even then it was a daily struggle, with the urge to drink always hanging over her. After six months, Gail brought up the other idea their counselor had mentioned.

"You know," said Gail, "I think you need to break free from this killer job you have. Admit it—despite how hard you're able to work, and despite the fact that the magazine is a feather in your cap—it's overwhelming and isn't going to get any better. You work all the time. We hardly have any relationship now."

Then Gail made a bold proposal. "I've been looking into teaching jobs in Upstate New York. With my experience in special education, I expect I can easily get a job, with maybe a small cut in salary but also smaller classes. The cost of living is also less there. I think I'd really like to pursue that. Plus I have the trust my grandparents left me with its annual payout. You know that I haven't really found something I wanted to spend that on—until now. How would you feel about asking your mother to join the bakery business? It's still going, right? And I know you'd be great at it—you could even grow the business. And I think you'd find it more satisfying than publishing. Do me a favor and just think about it."

Lila's ultimate solution for becoming a sober couple with Gail involved "coloring outside the lines," specifically the career change that Gail suggested. Lila took a good month to mull it over, along with many talks with Gail and their counselor, as well as with Lila's mother. But in the end, this unconventional solution proved to be the answer. Lila's lifestyle, she had to admit, was not that conducive to sobriety. There was simply no way to escape the ongoing, relentless stress. She faced a choice: continuing to be successful as a publisher, keeping her committed relationship with alcohol but losing the one with Gail, versus choosing a lifestyle that required hard work and commitment but also allowed for a life outside of work.

Her mother was thrilled when Lila expressed an interest in the bakery: "It will now be a third-generation bakery!" she pronounced, while adding the caution that Lila should not expect to get rich from it, at least not until the business expanded. Lila already had a few ideas about that, as customers had begun to request eat-in services as well as catering.

The solution that Lila and Gail opted for proved to be success-ful, and one year after their last counseling session, they were both happily sober in their new, chosen lifestyle. Of course, they were for-tunate in that they both had some savings to draw on, as well as Gail's solid career, her trust fund, and the fact that the bakery business was doing well. Not all couples have these advantages. Still, coloring outside the lines may help you as a couple navigate the pathway to becoming a sober couple. You and your partner should consider asking yourselves the following questions if you believe your sobriety journey may require some unconventional decisions:

- Do either one of you, after serious reflection and dialogue, believe that some aspect of your lifestyle together—like Lila's job—represents a serious, ongoing threat to becoming a sober couple? What is that threat?
- Do either one or both of you have a passion for something that you've never felt able to truly pursue, either because you didn't believe it was economically viable or because you believe it would somehow be disapproved of? What is that passion?
- If you decide to pursue that passion, what steps can you take to do so, on either a full- or part-time basis? Can you agree to support one another in such a pursuit, finding a way to make room for it in your lifestyle?

A LITMUS TEST FOR SOBER LOVE?

The reality is that simply deciding to pursue an identity as a sober couple in the context of living in a drinking culture does represent a diversion from the norm. People sometimes ask if there is some test or condition that is essential to the pursuit of sober love. If there is

such a test, it boils down to being committed to helping and supporting one another in a decision to pursue an identity as a sober couple.
Any ambivalence or reluctance in one or both partners is a recipe for
failure.

If one partner decides to pursue a sober identity and lifestyle but
the other responds negatively or with ambivalence to that idea, that
may be the kiss of death for sober love. In other words, if one partner decides that a sober identity is what they want but the other says,
"You can go ahead and stop drinking if you want to, but count me
out," or "It's your problem; I don't need to change," then sober love
may indeed be fated to die on the vine. That's why it is vital for couples
to reflect on and discuss their current identity, and whether they
might be up for the challenge of changing it. The following questions
may aid your discussions about the possibility of pursuing sober love:

- Where do you believe that each of you falls on the drinking
  spectrum? Is there a large disparity between you?
- How do each of you feel about the prospect of embracing an
  identity as a sober couple?
- How much of a role does *ambivalence* (discussed in chapter 6)
  play in any unwillingness either of you may have to let go of
  the drinking culture that you've been part of? Do you associate drinking with being "normal"?

If one of you is hesitant to change, you need to honestly ask yourself: How much am I willing to sacrifice in the interest of supporting
our relationship, as opposed to my personal preference? What is my
rationale for resisting? Believing that we will have to give up our social network? Fear of being labeled "abnormal"? Not wanting to give
up the experience of intoxication?

In any successful committed relationship, partners often have
to make changes and compromises in the interest of continuing the

relationship. Indeed, relationships sometimes require sacrifice in order to survive and thrive. This book acknowledges this reality and is intended to help couples save their relationship when drinking poses a threat to it.

If you and your partner find yourselves at different places on the drinking spectrum, then the issue of love may come into play, especially if one of you has a coherent, even compelling argument for pursuing a sober identity. In that case, the other partner needs to consider how much they are willing to sacrifice in the interest of the relationship, that third entity that bonds you together. That is often the true measure of sober love.

MOVING FORWARD

Few if any goals truly worth pursuing are likely to come easy. President John F. Kennedy, when announcing his decision to land a man on the moon within a decade, said, "We choose to go to the moon in this decade and do other things, not because they are easy, but because they are hard." The same could be said of a couple's decision to embrace a new identity as a sober couple, relying on love for one another and for their relationship to get them there. It's safe to say that every one of the abstinence-based fellowships cited in this book would agree that the pursuit of sobriety involves many challenges. After all, their very existence is an acknowledgment of this reality, while also seeing sober love as a goal worthy of shared commitment and persistence: that a sober life is better than a drinking life.

Chapter 13

BUMPS AND POTHOLES ON THE ROAD TO SOBER LOVE

PROGRESS, NOT PERFECTION

One common misperception that people have when it comes to fellowships like AA is that they demand total sobriety from their members. Some people who are unfamiliar with these fellowships even believe that a member will be "kicked out" if they have a drink. Nothing could be further from the truth, as all of these fellowships exist precisely because they recognize what a challenge sobriety can be. They provide the mutual support required to achieve and maintain that goal. Let's pause here to consider "progress, not perfection," which happens to be a phrase that readers who choose to join a fellowship as part of their recovery plan are likely to hear often.

Researchers like myself who have conducted rigorous research on the effectiveness of AA (the most ubiquitous but not the only fellowship supporting a sober lifestyle) are faced with the following questions: How do we define success when evaluating the effectiveness of a fellowship in promoting a sober lifestyle? Is 100% sobriety the best measure? Does that correspond to reality? The answer is no.

Your goal as a couple, of course, is sobriety. That said, does it follow that you should seek only perfection, while ignoring significant progress along the way? I think not. In similar fashion, researchers assessing the effectiveness of treatments for drinking problems have naturally looked at total abstinence as one measure of success. But they have been inclined to also embrace progress over perfection when assessing a therapeutic intervention, using the following measures.

Percentage of Days Abstinent (PDA): Men and women in treatment report how many days they were able to be sober over a specific period, such as 30, 60, or 90 days. Researchers also ask how many days these individuals were sober prior to entering treatment, leading to two PDA scores, before treatment versus during or after treatment. If a person's PDA before treatment was, say, only 10% but increased to 85% after several weeks of treatment, that would be considered a measure of success. Similarly, if 85% of a group of individuals reported being sober throughout that period, that would also be considered a sign of successful treatment.

Drinks per Drinking Day (PDD): Researchers are interested in learning not only how many days the people they treat are sober, but also how much they drink if they have a slip. This is where PDD comes in. If a person drank once in the past 30 days and had two drinks, that would be a measure of progress as compared to having six drinks. It's also more in line with the real-life experience of people who choose to pursue a sober lifestyle, or the idea of *recovery, which is best thought of as an ongoing process as opposed to an event.* In other words, individuals do not typically move from misusing alcohol to abstinence in one single step.

Progress, not perfection is a helpful framework for couples pursuing sober love. Couples considering sobriety can ask themselves, *How are we doing?* As you take stock of how far you've come in achieving your goal, both individually and as a couple, this very idea of progress, not perfection tends to permeate the culture of fellowships that seek to promote the same goal. While I do not advocate simply sweeping slips under the proverbial rug, I believe it's important to "accentuate the positive," as a song by Aretha Franklin advises us.

TAKING STOCK

When discussing just how far you as a couple have come so far in your pursuit of becoming a sober couple, take some time to take stock of the following:

- *Percentage of Days Abstinent*: Over the past 60 days, how many of those days were each of you able to not have a drink? All of them? If so, give yourselves a pat on the back. If one of you did drink, how many times? Does any difference between you reflect some ambivalence that one of you has about becoming a sober couple? What is the percentage of sober days you as a couple have been able to accumulate over the past 60 days? How does that compare with the amount of sober days you would have typically had in the past?

- *Drinks per Drinking Day*: If one (or both) of you did drink, how many drinks did you consume, and how does that compare to how many drinks you would likely have had on a similar day in the past? Do you see any progress here, or do you tend to fall back to where you were when you do drink? If it was just one of you, how did your partner react? On a scale of 1 (not at all) to 10 (very much), how motivated are you to increase your percentage of days abstinent and reduce your drinks per drinking day?

- *Renovations*: All of the couples described in this book made some significant "renovations" to their lifestyle in order to support their goal of becoming a sober couple. What renovations did you decide upon? How well have you followed through on these plans? Have they helped? Is there anything else you'd like to add to your renovation plan?

- *Shared Pleasures*: Has drinking begun to shrink or "hollow out" your relationship? What shared pleasures gradually fell by the wayside? Are there any that you would like to recover, and if so, how much progress have you made? Do you have any ideas for new shared pleasures that you would be interested in pursuing? Have a conversation and list a few shared pleasures that you would like to pursue. Be sure to describe how you will fit these into your lifestyle.
- *Manageability*: Are there any ways in which your lifestyle as a couple became less manageable as drinking played a larger part in your lives? What have the effects of drinking been on the following?
  - Overall physical health and fitness
  - Financial stability
  - Work life
  - Family life
  - Have you seen improvements in any of these areas as a result of pursuing a sober lifestyle?

Taking the time to do an inventory of your relationship like the above can accomplish two things. First, it can help you to identify and accentuate the positives you may have experienced so far. Second, it can guide you to the areas you'd like to work on a bit more as a couple moving forward. I strongly encourage you to do this periodically.

THE ROAD TO SOBER LOVE

As pointed out above, fellowships that support those wanting a sober lifestyle recognize that the road to sober love is not likely to be free from bumps and even potholes along the way. Let's now look at some of the complicating factors that couples are wise to keep in mind as they travel this road.

SOBRIETY AND FAMILY CULTURE

In chapter 4, we discussed what it takes to succeed at the goal of be-coming a sober couple, including the concept of *psychological hardi-ness*. This characteristic has been linked to better physical and mental health. One of the qualities associated with hardiness is the belief, to again invoke our analogy, that life is not a smooth road but is rather marked by occasional hazards. To expect things to be easy makes a person vulnerable to anxiety, hopelessness, and depression. To-gether, hardiness and sober love—plus a deep commitment to each other and their relationship—can help couples successfully navigate "troubled waters."

Before we look at a few of these challenges, let's pause to take stock of just what your attitude is toward life in general. I encourage you as a couple to reflect on and discuss the follow-ing questions about how your families dealt with life's ups and downs:

- Families tend to develop a culture of their own. Did your family teach that if a person worked hard and followed the rules, then life should be relatively easy? Or was your family culture accepting of the idea that life can be smooth some-times and bumpy at other times, regardless of how hard a person works or how good they are?
- How did your family react in times of crisis, such as a parent losing a job or a loved one being diagnosed with a serious ill-ness? Did they rise to the challenge calmly, or did they react with great anxiety—as though it was unfair or, worse, that they were helpless victims of life?
- Did your family pull together in the face of a crisis, or did the crisis pull them apart?

- Would you describe your family as being generally optimistic or pessimistic?
- Has either of you absorbed your family's attitude toward life? Would you say that attitude reflects psychological fragility or psychological hardiness? Are you ever caught by surprise when life throws you a curve ball, or do you more or less take it in stride?
- Are you as a couple inclined to pull together in the face of a challenge, or do you tend to withdraw from one another?

Despite your family culture and background, psychological hardiness is something you can work on and change. That's because it is at its essence an *attitude*, and attitudes can change. People are not always conscious of how their attitudes toward life reflect the family culture they were raised in. They more or less unconsciously absorb these attitudes, as opposed to consciously choosing them. They are not, for example, aware of how their family culture may have advocated caution over risk-taking, or security and predictability over adventure, or of pessimism over optimism. Some families value predictability, conformity, and risk avoidance above all else, while other families are more comfortable with the idea of individuality—of pursuing "a road less taken."

When it comes to contemplating a new identity as a sober couple, certain attitudes will help set you up for success, especially in the context of living in a drinking culture (and in a family that may well be part of that drinking culture). Changing an attitude that stands in the way of sober love is possible, but it helps to have both insight and support: insight into the influence that an individual's family culture may play in their willingness to face a challenge, plus support along the way.

Having insight into the role your respective family cultures may play in your attitudes toward life in general (and sober love in particular) can be a springboard for change. That's because insight opens the door to action. But change also typically requires ongoing encouragement and support. The most important source of that support is your relationship with your partner. Additional support may come from a recovery fellowship or a counselor who plays a similar role. The choice of course is yours. You or your partner may decide that you need both a fellowship and a counselor to help you with your goal of sobriety.

SELF-CONFIDENCE

Another factor that plays a decisive role in realizing an identity as a sober couple may sound simple but it is powerful, and that is self-confidence, or what psychologists like to call *self-efficacy*. This boils down to the idea that you have what it takes to succeed, and it too is often part of a family's "culture."

Self-confidence (self-efficacy) includes a belief that the skills you already have, plus the skills you believe you can learn, will enable you to survive a crisis or achieve a goal. Families' cultures also differ on this dimension, with some embracing a positive, optimistic self-efficacy attitude, and others being prone to feelings of hopelessness and helplessness, especially in the face of crisis. As one colleague put it to me, "My family's attitude was always that disaster was just around the corner, and that the best we could do was hunker down and hope to minimize the damage." He felt that this attitude had come to dominate his outlook on life, though for a long time he had not truly recognized it for what it was and how it had affected him. Eventually, he came to recognize his family's collective fear of new things and reticence to take on challenges. His family members were inclined to hold on to security, even when that security stood in the way of advancement or a better lifestyle. For a long time, he'd just written this off to conservatism, but eventually he came to see it as fear and a collective lack of self-confidence or self-efficacy.

When facing the challenge of becoming a sober couple, it's obvious what role psychological hardiness and self-efficacy can play in the outcome. The fact is that the family culture we grow up within does tend to exert an influence on how we approach life and its inevitable challenges. Even some objectively successful people can attest to being inwardly wary, much like my colleague, that disaster lies just around the corner or that they will be overwhelmed by a crisis at some point. Such thinking contributes to a sort of "freefloating anxiety" that hovers over them like a cloud. At times it can stand in the way of facing a challenge, like becoming a sober couple. It may seem like a goal that is simply impossible.

If either (or both) of you can identify with an outlook of psychological fragility or a lack of self-efficacy, the good news is that this insight can be a springboard to change. Moreover, you can be one another's best friend when it comes to supporting that change. But first you must recognize to what extent this life view characterized your family culture. If you can, think of and share with your partner a couple of examples when a crisis, either big or small, evoked anxiety and pessimism. Then ponder and share some examples of when you adopted an optimistic attitude, a confidence that the crisis could be managed. Such self-confidence can play a crucial role in supporting sober love despite any challenges along the way.

BERT AND STACY

Bert and Stacy had been in a relationship for just shy of a year, having met through an online dating app for people over 40. In their profiles, both stated that they were social drinkers, though the truth was that both had a significant relationship with drinking. Stacy was the mother of a grown daughter who lived several hours away and was attending law school part time while working as a teacher's aide.

Stacy had been divorced for five years. Over that period she had fallen into a social life that included a number of heavy-drinking friends. Though in the past she'd had friends who either did not drink or drank at a low-risk level, her current group consisted mostly of women around her age whose lifestyle included meeting at a local pub for drinks and dinner twice a week. On these occasions, there was as much if not more drinking than eating. Stacy would often drive home from these meet-ups with a blood alcohol level that put her over the legal limit, but so far she had gotten away with driving while intoxicated. She did not drink as much on other weeknights, though there was rarely a night when she did not drink at all. On weekends, she would typically start drinking in the late afternoon with one or two glasses of wine.

For his part, Bert had begun to recognize, at least privately, that his relationship with drinking had evolved to the point where it was just that—a "relationship"—though he didn't consciously use that word. He could admit, however, that based on his habit of drinking two or more cocktails every night (bourbon on ice being his favorite), along with an increasing tendency to fall asleep while watching TV on his lounge chair by nine o'clock, was not the lifestyle he ideally wanted. Also divorced, Bert had a grown son who had recently married and was hoping to start a family of his own.

A talented engineer, Bert was employed as a lead design professional for a growing environmental technology firm. Though well paid for his expertise, his workload in recent years had increased steadily, with no additional help being offered despite his asking for it several times. That was then complicated by the fact that his work often included time spent consulting with potential customers to discuss their needs, including after-hours entertaining, such as business dinners that almost always involved drinks. He was aware that his drinking had definitely increased alongside the added workload, the associated stress, and a social network that promoted drinking. To make matters worse, he felt that he had lost some of the vigor with which he had previously approached his work. He wasn't sure that anyone else had noticed his decreased vitality, but what mattered was that he did, and he believed it could eventually show up in his job performance, if it hadn't already.

When they first started dating, neither Bert nor Stacy was interested in talking about their drinking habits. But on their third date, Stacy drank enough that Bert insisted on calling and paying for an Uber to take her home (even though he, too, had enough to be considered intoxicated). A week later they met again, and Stacy apologized for her drinking. Bert waved her apology away and then told her that he too would have gotten a DUI if he'd been pulled over on the way home that night. He then took a step further and said that he thought he might have "a little drinking problem" and had even considered stopping, at least for a while.

Bert's admission opened the door for Stacy to share. She admitted that she thought she might be drinking "a little too much lately" as well. They left it at that for the moment, but on their next date a couple of weeks later, Bert brought up his own drinking again. Since their previous date, his doctor had said that the results of his last annual physical suggested that he was a candidate for eventual diabetes. Bert had been worried ever since. He had a brother who was diabetic, as was his mother, and their conditions limited them significantly. He shared with Stacy that he had decided not to have more than a single cocktail on any day, including on their dates.

Stacy told Bert that she understood and respected his decision. But she then proceeded to have three drinks on their next date, while he had just one, and this time Bert insisted on driving her home. This led to a crisis in this incubating relationship. On the one hand, Bert and Stacy found that they had much in common, including grown children, successful careers (hers as a realtor), shared values, and even common interests they'd each once enjoyed but had largely both abandoned thanks to their respective relationships with alcohol. These lost pleasures included taking easy hikes, visiting county fairs, watching vintage movies, trying out different kinds of cuisine, and listening to live jazz music. They were also physically attracted to one another, and conversations between them went smoothly. But the bottom line was that Bert had to admit that his ability to stick to one cocktail had been difficult, especially during their dates. His resolve was likely to be severely tested if Stacy chose to continue drinking as much as she did. She said she would have to think about whether she could curtail her drinking when they were together, and they left it at that.

The next evening, Stacy called Bert and told him that she'd had a chance to think about their last conversation. On reflection, she realized that her own drinking had definitely increased since her divorce, and mostly in the context of the new social network she'd settled into. She thought that at least one of her friends might have a "drinking problem," but Stacy was not sure that she'd label any of them as alcoholics. She didn't think she was an alcoholic either, but she did admit that she seemed to have difficulty on those social occasions limiting herself to one drink. "I'm okay with not drinking at all at home at times, or having just one glass of wine," she explained, "but I realize now that once I start drinking with friends, I do drink too much." She had decided that she was going to tell her drinking friends that would be quitting "for a while" in the interest of her health, as her mother and sister both had recently been treated for cancer. Stacy added that it was okay with her if Bert decided to stick with his one drink limit, but that she was not going to drink at all when they were together, at least for now.

Stacy and Bert's relationship entered a new chapter after Stacy's decision. As it turned out, she was indeed able to not drink at all when they were together, and she even decided, for the time being, to eliminate the wine she drank at home during the week as well. Somewhat to her surprise, she felt much better being sober. "I guess I'd gotten so used to drinking a few times a week that I didn't appreciate how it was affecting me. But I really do like being sober," she shared with Bert.

Unfortunately, Bert's experience was different, in part because of his different history. Stacy reported that no one in her family had what she could call a drinking problem. Not that they didn't drink—but they were what she described as "social drinkers." Alcohol—mostly beer and wine—was always available at family functions, but she could not recall any family member ever drinking to excess or getting drunk. Nor were there any rumors about family members with drinking problems that she could recall. Her own increased drinking, then, appeared to be correlated primarily with her divorce and the subsequent new social network she'd settled into.

Bert's story was very different. He'd started drinking—mostly beer—in high school, and had never really stopped drinking since, through college, graduate school, and then in his career. Despite his heavy drinking, he'd been successful professionally. He did acknowledge that his drinking had played a role in his marital problems (in particular, sexual dysfunction and less time spent talking and interacting with one another), but he maintained that he'd always been a good provider and a source of steady support for his son. His own family included a long line of men who, as he described it, were known for their ability to "hold their liquor." As a young man he'd more or less taken pride in that—as well as his capacity to drink without passing out like some of his college friends. On looking back, he could see now how that might have been more of a curse than a blessing. He eventually shared with a counselor he'd begun seeing how he'd always suspected (although it was never discussed within the family) that his maternal grandfather had died of cirrhosis of the liver.

Bert met again with Stacy and this time laid his cards on the table. He really liked her, he said, more than any woman he'd dated since his divorce. He enjoyed doing things with Stacy, including some of those shared pleasures that he'd abandoned over time but was experiencing again with her, as well as just how generally comfortable he felt with her. Stacy told him that the feelings were mutual. Then she asked him how he was doing with his one-drink policy, and he had to admit that it had not been going well. When out with her he could stick to one drink, but at home by himself, he'd drink several glasses of bourbon on the rocks, and he was still prone to falling asleep in his lounge chair as opposed to his bed. That was true even after he'd been with her and had only one cocktail. On arriving home those nights, the first thing he'd do was pour a drink. Moreover, on several recent occasions when he'd entertained prospective or current business clients over dinner, he'd had several drinks, usually along with them. "There's no question I was drunk," he told Stacy, "though I doubt the clients could tell, especially since most of them drank as much or more than I did, thanks to my company picking up the tab."

SOLUTIONS

I'll leave it up to the reader to decide whether Stacy and Bert's experiences were examples of what you might call hitting a bump in the road, versus running into a dangerous pothole. Either way, they had very different experiences exploring sobriety together. Stacy did not have the long history of drinking that Bert did. Her drinking, while surely heavy at times, was mostly limited to a social context. She did drink at home, but not every day and not nearly as much as she did when she was at a pub with her drinking friends. Bert, in contrast, did have a long history of nearly continuous drinking. He came from a family in which the men at least appeared to have a strong tolerance for alcohol—much to their disadvantage—and where some may have paid a heavy medical price for their drinking. Moreover, in contrast to Stacy, Bert drank heavily at home, daily, and his lifestyle, including his habits and routines, had significantly changed so as to accommodate drinking over time.

To their credit, both of them recognized what connected them to one another, and they valued their relationship as something worthy of nurturing. Neither one was willing to simply let that go, and both were able to admit that they did not truly enjoy the drinking life they'd settled into. So, the challenge that faced them now was how to pursue their relationship with sobriety as its basis—how to become a *sober couple* in the context of a drinking culture.

Bert and Stacy pursued their respective (but shared) challenges in different but appropriate ways. Most importantly, they now had a shared goal and supported one another in pursuing it.

Stacy opted to simply tell her friends that she'd decided to stop drinking for health reasons, without offering any specific period of sobriety. In addition, she sought to widen her social circle to include women who either didn't drink at all or drank only on rare social occasions. It turned out she knew plenty of such women but had drifted away from them as her lifestyle had come to accommodate drinking. Little by little, she reached out to and reconnected with a few of them.

Bert's challenge required something more. His first step was to meet with his doctor, ostensibly to discuss his potential for developing diabetes. Once there, though, he shared the real issue on his mind: his heavy drinking. The doctor spent some time with Bert going over some medical options, including a couple of medications. The doctor also recommended that Bert seek counseling, as well as try out AA or another recovery fellowship. Bert replied that he was in counseling and had a partner who was pursuing the same goal (sobriety). He said he was willing to consider the fellowship idea, though he also wanted to explore the medication option. He added that he was also in the process of making some modifications to his lifestyle.

On reviewing several different medication options that might help him stay sober, Bert told his doctor that he preferred the most aggressive option. This was Disulfiram, a medication he'd need to take every day, which would result in a severe negative reaction (nausea or vomiting) if he drank. Bert told his doctor he preferred this "no-nonsense" option over medication that might only reduce his urge to drink. He was "a grown man," he explained, who'd missed an opportunity to change his drinking habits years earlier. "Now I'm in a battle with the booze," he said, "and I may be losing it. It's threatening my health, and it may very well threaten my relationship." The doctor replied that he was on board with Bert's decision.

Bert also made the following renovations to his lifestyle:

- He eliminated all liquor from his condo. In couples counseling sessions with Stacy, Bart admitted that getting rid of all the alcohol at home had been difficult. The counselor suggested he write a goodbye letter to bourbon. They both laughed at that, though Bert ended up writing the letter and sharing it with the counselor.
- He removed the lounge chair from his family room and replaced it with an antique wooden rocking chair that had

been a family heirloom. Although comfortable, the rocking chair was not conducive to falling asleep.

- He let his son know that he'd decided to stop drinking—a decision his son fully supported.
- He regularly called his son three evenings to check in, instead of pouring a drink.
- He and Stacy started memberships at a new fitness center. They went together twice a week for some relatively easy exercise, followed by a healthy light dinner at home.
- He made a point of seeking out weekend venues for live music, usually preceded by (a sober) dinner at a new restaurant.
- He met Stacy on Sunday mornings for an easy hike or a visit to a local flea market, followed by a hearty breakfast.

An even more dramatic renovation in his lifestyle happened when Bert decided to approach the human resources department of his company. He'd done some research and learned that many companies were now excluding liquor costs from expense accounts for business entertaining. Without disclosing his own issue, Bert explained that he felt that some customers took advantage of the fact that they could drink on the company's dime when he took them out for lunch or dinner. He said he did not see this as a necessary expense, and cited the trend he'd discovered. A week later, the company issued an email clarifying the policy on expense accounts and stated that alcoholic drinks were not allowed expenses. Starting then, Bert politely told customers that he was happy to pay for their lunch or dinner, but they would need to pay for any alcoholic drinks. Bert immediately noticed a dramatic decrease in the number of drinks his clients ordered. As a result, he found it relatively easy to avoid ordering a drink for himself.

MOVING FORWARD

After a year and a half, Bert and Stacy were still a sober couple and enjoying it. Both said they were amazed at how much more energy they had, and how much richer their lifestyle together was now as compared to what it had been as two drinking individuals. In counseling, Bert added (with a smile) that the intermittent sexual dysfunction that had dogged him for years was no longer a problem.

Chapter 14

SLIPPING AND SLIDING

IN DISCUSSING THE LYRICS to his song "Slip Slidin' Away," Paul Simon explained that they refer to what can happen if we don't live deliberately—just existing without purpose or direction. That pretty much sums up what it's like to simply go along with the drinking culture and allow alcohol to occupy an increasing part of your lifestyle. And as the couples highlighted in this book have shown, life can become much more mutually fulfilling as a sober couple. If you doubt that, visit some of the sources that I've referenced (included in the appendix), and read what individuals (and by extension, couples) have to say about sober living.

The further an individual or couple moves along the drinking spectrum over time, the more likely it is that goals they have (or shared at one time) may begin to slip away. This slow deterioration is evident in the stories shared in this book. That being said, it's important to allow for the possibility of the occasional "slip" or "slide" along the way, as it is unrealistic to expect a totally smooth road to sobriety. This chapter addresses these normal lapses, giving couples tools to face them and help reduce the chances of a slip happening again.

Everyone knows (or should know) that despite the best intentions, plans often go awry. In fact, anyone who has attempted to give up something, or some activity, that has become woven into the fabric of their lifestyle knows how difficult it can be to avoid either a momentary slip, or even a prolonged slide. That is true whether it's alcohol, or chocolate, or ice cream, or even a so-called healthy addiction, like running or lifting weights. In other words, setbacks are to be expected on the road to becoming a sober couple, just as they were when Kennedy challenged the nation to send a man to the moon. With that in mind, it's imperative that you know what to do if a slip or slide does occur. And rest assured, if it does, you will have plenty of individuals and couples who can relate to your situation.

In chapter 13 we discussed the idea of how to measure success in the pursuit of pursuing an identity as a sober couple. Guidelines for taking stock of how a couple could realistically assess their success along the way were presented there as well. In this chapter, we move on to a more granular look at the issue of slips. The fact of the matter is that one or both partners are likely to experience one.

Slips, even full relapses (a return to prior drinking), should not be cause for despair, but neither should they be quickly dismissed. A simple "I'm okay now" following a slip into drinking could set the stage for a lengthy relapse by falsely implying that there's nothing to worry about. It may be tempting to seek solace in such an attitude, but it is dangerous thinking.

It is fairly common to attribute a slip to what is called a "craving," or a physical desire to have a drink. Such cravings are real, and they can occur on a conscious level during the day or in the form of dreams. Recovery fellowships advise members to turn to the fellowship for support in order to either talk through or distract themselves from a craving. In fact, being able to be open about a craving ("sitting on a drink," in AA parlance) is considered a sign of strength, not weakness.

But there is another, less obvious but no less dangerous way that slips may be triggered. An analogy would be to think about the computer you probably own. When using your computer, you are no doubt aware of programs that you are running in the "foreground," such as a word processor. But there are also programs that simultaneously run in the "background," which you may not be aware of.

Let's turn now to examining how a slip (drinking) can be caused by something running more or less in the background of your consciousness. It may not occur to you the role that such forces can play in triggering "that first drink." But these factors can be analyzed in response to a slip, so as to enlighten couples as to what might need to change to prevent another slip moving forward. In many cases, this may mean what might need to be avoided. There are three contexts or dimensions that define a slip: the *cognitive* context, the *social* context, and the *emotional* context. We will examine each of them as well as what they can teach us.

THE COGNITIVE CONTEXT OF SLIPS

The cognitive context of slips can be summed up with a question: "What were you thinking at the time of your slip?" This brings us back to an important previous discussion, about what each individual truly believes about his or her drinking. Specifically, have they thought it through and concluded that it's in the best interest of them as individuals and as a couple to become sober? Alternatively, is either (or both) of them *ambivalent* about this? We looked at research on moderation and so-called controlled use, as well as what difference a person's goal makes for their chances of recovery. That research informs us that those men and women whose drinking places them at least in the moderate zone on the drinking spectrum, and who choose abstinence over controlled use, have the best outcomes. For these men and women, research on moderation and controlled use shows poor results at best. Nevertheless, despite these realities, many programs and practitioners promise success with moderation. It can be tempting to consider moderation, playing into the ambivalence that undermines a commitment to becoming a sober couple.

A second thought process that often plays a role in slips is *complacency*. If you recall from chapter 3, Jake convinced himself that after a couple of weeks of not drinking, he "deserved" a martini. No doubt he thought he could now control his drinking. That complacency quickly led back to where he'd started: square in the middle of the moderate drinking zone, with his wife feeling betrayed.

If one or both of you experience a slip and return to drinking (even on one occasion), have a talk about whether abstinence is still the best goal to pursue as a couple, versus holding on to the notion that drinking is controllable. People who utilize AA as a means of support to stay sober like to describe alcoholism as a "cunning disease," one that tells you that you don't have it. Whether you are inclined to think of problem drinking as a disease in the strictly medical sense, or as a behavior that is influenced by multiple factors as described in this book, the fact is that both ambivalence and complacency remain prime suspects when it comes to slippin' and slidin'.

When assessing the cognitive context of a slip, the following questions may prove helpful:

- When you slipped or slid back into drinking, what were you thinking? Were you motivated in part by ambivalence or complacency?
- What was your goal at that point: controlled drinking or sobriety?
- What is your thinking now about becoming a sober couple?

JEREMY

Jeremy is an example of just how dangerous ambivalence and complacency can be. Just 20 years old and a college junior, he was hospitalized following a college party where he drank so much that he passed out and nearly choked on his own vomit. His fellow partiers dialed 911, and emergency medical technicians gave Jeremy oxygen and prepared an automated exterior defibrillator (AED) in case he went into cardiac arrest. They then took him by ambulance to the hospital.

It turned out that drinking this heavily was not an unusual event for Jeremy. On arrival at the hospital, doctors determined that his alcohol blood level was dangerously close to the poisonous level, and that his life could be in danger. For two days he stayed in the hospital, at which point his parents picked him up and drove directly to a rehab facility. Jeremy spent the next two weeks there, attending several group therapy sessions daily and participating in AA meetings.

Jeremy's heavy drinking had started even before high school. He described himself as extremely gregarious but also insecure, about his physique and attractiveness (he was rather slender) as well as about his intelligence. He attributed his ability to socialize in large part to the large amounts of alcohol he would drink before parties. In that inebriated state he was able to talk, joke, and get along with his peers—who generally couldn't tell he was drunk. Once at a party, he'd continue to drink. He was even able to flirt with women he found attractive, though he'd never had a steady girlfriend.

In treatment, Jeremy admitted that he had a drinking problem, that it was bad, and that it was dangerous. But when he attended the AA meetings and therapy groups in rehab, he sometimes doubted that he was "as bad as others" who told stories of even worse consequences associated with drinking. After discharge, with an appointment with a therapist for follow-up, Jeremy was able to abstain from drinking for three months. One problem, however, was that he did not socialize at all with friends during that time. He stayed with his parents and drove to classes for the remainder of that semester. He did talk to some friends via cellphone and texts, but otherwise he remained socially isolated. The thought of accepting an invitation to socialize brought on anxiety, so he made excuses, including the truth—that he'd decided to quit drinking "for a while."

After nearly three months of sobriety, Jeremy was feeling physically well and energetic, but he was also bored. He gladly helped out around his parents' home and had picked up his old hobbies of nature photography and rebuilding old stereo equipment. He chose not to try a fellowship (though his therapist had suggested either AA or SMART Recovery), and his nights had become increasingly uncomfortable. Then one day a female friend, Gretchen, whom Jeremy had something of a crush on, called. She had heard about Jeremy's decision to stop drinking, and she supported that decision. She added that she had no expectation of his drinking around her, and that she could also abstain if that would help. Then she said that she was planning a Fourth of July party and hoped that Jeremy would come. He replied that he'd think about it and let her know.

Jeremy ended up attending the party, where he gave into temptation and accepted a drink. Through the course of the party, one drink became six, along with a few shots of tequila. When Gretchen asked if he was okay, Jeremy laughed. "Sure!" he said, though Gretchen could see that he was drunk. She ended up driving him home, where she dropped him off with his clearly concerned parents waiting at the door.

The cognitive context of Jeremy's slide was both ambivalence and complacency. He told himself that it would be safe for him to go to the party because, first, Gretchen said that she understood that he was not drinking and, second, he had nearly three months of sobriety under his belt. That thinking proved to be Michael's undoing. Here's why:

- Even though Jeremy had been sober for nearly three months, he had developed a false sense of confidence (complacency) that he was immune from his long-standing habit of heavy drinking in social situations. The problem was not in Jeremy's intentions, but rather in the false sense of safety he'd settled into.
- Jeremy had done little, other than a couple of brief conversations with his therapist, to address his true ambivalence about the severity of his drinking and the need to be sober as opposed to trying to control his drinking. Naturally, ambivalence won out as soon as he arrived at Gretchen's party.
- Though Gretchen had said she could avoid drinking, she had no control over Jeremy when a male friend offered him a beer. Jeremy accepted after telling himself, *I'll have just one.*

The cognitive context of Jeremy's slip (and its potential for a full slide into addiction) is a common one. In other words, what he was thinking had a direct impact on his actions. As is common in many slides, he told himself that it would be "safe" (perhaps because he had three months of sobriety, or perhaps Gretchen was there) to have a drink.

Ambivalence and complacency like Jeremy's operate almost subconsciously, like a program running in the background of your computer. That's why it is so important to have an honest conversation with your partner about where you each fall on the drinking spectrum and what you can to do avoid a slip.

THE SOCIAL CONTEXT OF SLIPS

Whereas the cognitive context of a slip has to do with what a person was thinking, the social context has to do with *where they were and who they were with*. Oftentimes the cognitive and social contexts overlap, though it's helpful to consider each one independently. In the case of Jeremy's slip, this overlap is obvious. Not only did he tell himself he could safely have a drink, but he did so while at a party with peers who drank.

There are also instances where the social context is the dominant influence. There are couples, for example, who decide to become a sober couple, only to find themselves (either unintentionally or deliberately) in a situation, and among people, who support the very drinking that they had vowed to avoid. One common example—discussed in chapter 13—has to do with family. It's no secret that substance use disorder runs in families, be that for genetic or social reasons. Regardless, the bottom line is that despite their acceptance of the need to be sober, a couple may find it difficult to avoid having a drink in certain social situations that include family members who drink. Let's look at one couple who faced this problem.

MITCH AND GREG

The youngest of three sons, Mitch was raised by a father who had a strong work ethic and was a good provider, but he worked two jobs and was often absent. Mitch's mother was an alcoholic whose drinking problem was plain as day but never discussed within the family. She drank every day, and it was not unusual for Mitch to find her passed out in bed when he got home from school. It was often up to him and his two sisters to take care of the household. Both parents had siblings, so family gatherings tended to be large, raucous affairs with a great deal of drinking. Mitch knew (though it was never talked about) that several family members, including aunts, uncles, and cousins, also had drinking problems.

Of the three children, Mitch's oldest sister went on to finish only high school due largely to her own drinking. She married young as a means of gaining some independence, had a child, and settled into a low-income family life. His other sister also left home at age 18, to work full time while attending community college, and from there became a dental assistant. She eventually moved to another state, where she now lived with another woman.

As for Mitch, objectively you could say that he was the most successful child, in that he went to college and then on to graduate school, eventually working as a financial adviser for a large firm. His clients liked him, and over time he'd built a significant and loyal client base that made his job both enjoyable and secure. He'd had two relationships, each of which had lasted over two years, but both of them had ended, one because his partner had decided to pursue a job opportunity abroad (which Mitch felt he could not accommodate, given his own career), and one when the man proposed marriage but Mitch realized that he did not love him or their relationship that much.

Along the way, Mitch, like his mother, began drinking more and more. He had an epiphany after experiencing a blackout at a party that alcohol had become too much a part of his life and looked up an alcohol counselor. After an initial assessment, the counselor agreed that Mitch fit the criteria for a diagnosis of severe alcohol use disorder. They discussed moderation, but when Mitch talked about his mother, and in light of the blackout, the counselor advocated quitting altogether, to avoid a repetition of his mother's fate as well as more severe consequences.

Mitch also met with his doctor, who supported the decision to abstain. He also recommended that Mitch start taking Vivitrol, an injectable medication to help reduce any cravings for alcohol. Between his own decision to stop, the support of a counselor, and medication, Mitch was able to achieve sobriety. A year later he was feeling well physically. He'd lost ten pounds and improved his conditioning by joining a gym. By then he had also started dating Greg, who he felt might be someone he'd want to commit to, if things progressed in that direction. Greg was a drinker, however. He did not drink excessively, but he did drink regularly, mainly in social situations but also at home to the tune of a couple of glasses of wine two or three nights a week. Greg knew that Mitch chose to be sober, but Mitch initially avoided the issue of being sober together.

Mitch stuck with his therapy sessions, and during that first year of sobriety, he was able to avoid face-to-face contact with his family, keeping in touch through phone calls and emails. But then the issue of his parents' fiftieth anniversary came up. His sister said that she felt obligated to plan a celebration, one that would include everyone in the extended family. The problem for Mitch, though, was that he knew that his mother was not the only family member who drank, and he was sure that any anniversary celebration would mean lots of alcohol on hand. Mitch then had a decision to make: Would he go to the party?

Mitch's dilemma is typical of how social context can contribute to a slip. Some people may intentionally place themselves in such risky situations, intending to stay sober and thinking that they will be safe because of their good intentions. (Consider the gambling addict who says he likes going to a casino because the restaurants are good.) Too often, even the best intentions present a false hope. In Mitch's case, however, he had the advantage of knowing in advance that the anniversary celebration presented a risky situation. On the one hand, he was confident in his sobriety, and committed to it, even when he was with Greg. On the other hand, he knew he was vulnerable to situations that could tempt his resolve, especially if Greg chose to drink.

Mitch spoke with his counselor, and in the end they decided that Mitch had three viable choices: go to the party with Greg and risk drinking; go to the party with Greg, stay close, and ask him to refrain from drinking, then leave early; or just not go.

In the end, Mitch opted to ask Greg if he was willing to go to the family party, not drink, and leave early. That worked. It also set the stage for a discussion about their relationship, and whether Greg was up for considering being a sober couple if they were to move toward commitment. At the time of this writing, that issue has not been fully decided, though their relationship is still going strong.

Couples may find the following guide helpful in discussing the social context of slips:

- Take some time to identify (preferably in advance) situations and places where the risk of using alcohol is maximal. Often these will include social gatherings with friends, coworkers, or family.
- Next, identify places and situations where the risk of drinking is minimal. Activities such as working out, running, hiking, and playing tennis may fit this bill. Or they may include going to alternative types of social places, like museums, craft fairs, or healthy restaurants. Perhaps these include social interactions with others who choose not to drink. Finally, consider the idea of an abstinence-based fellowship as a social "safe harbor" that supports a sober lifestyle.
- Take an honest inventory of those social situations that have been associated with drinking in the past, along with ones that are likely to be (like Mitch's parents' anniversary party) in the future. Brainstorm about whether to attend, and if so, how to

attend without endangering your commitment to being a sober couple. Can a partner, like Greg, play a role in dealing with them? Better yet, if both partners are working on building a sober lifestyle, can they rely on each other to successfully negotiate such challenging situations?

THE EMOTIONAL CONTEXT OF SLIPS

Thus far we have covered two of the three contexts that are associated with slips and slides. These are "What were you thinking?" and "Where were you and who were you with?" To complete the analysis of a slip, we also need to consider a third question: "What were you feeling?"

If a couple newly committed to a sober identity can answer these questions, they will have a leg up on avoiding slip slidin' away moving forward. To answer this third question, it's important to identify those emotions that are most often associated with alcohol use, mostly as a way of coping. These emotions may make individuals vulnerable to drinking, a situation that can escalate over time.

ANXIETY

Men and women have long turned to alcohol in an effort to self-medicate anxiety. In low doses (low-risk drinking), alcohol can actually help to reduce anxiety. One glass of wine before a social event can help a shy person overcome their social anxiety enough to be able to socialize. As the expression goes, a little alcohol in these situations helps a shy person "come out of their shell." The problem is that for people whose genetic makeup includes the ability to build a tolerance to alcohol over time, as well as those whose social networks promote drinking, one glass of wine (or one cocktail) can easily progress to two, three, or more. At that point, alcohol ceases to have a calming effect and begins to have a depressive effect. That depression, mild as it might be, often leads to even more drinking. And so the pathway opens to an alcohol use disorder.

Anxiety disorders, like alcohol use disorders, tend to run in families, and they may reflect a genetic vulnerability. Anxiety may also be part of another disorder, such as posttraumatic stress disorder (PTSD). One of the symptoms of PTSD is what psychologists call "free-floating anxiety," or anxiety that seems to have no objective source but lingers over an individual like a cloud. For those who are burdened with PTSD, drinking can actually worsen free-floating anxiety.

People who suffer from chronic anxiety can be ashamed to admit it, as though it's a character defect. But if an individual or couple can recognize anxiety as something that motivates them to drink, as well as where and when it comes into play most strongly, they can use that insight to explore alternative ways of dealing with it. For example, those who have been subject to sexual abuse, either as children or adults, will often experience anxiety in any situation that triggers a memory (even an unconscious one) of the circumstances associated with their abuse. Making this connection can open the door to learning how to minimize that response without alcohol.

Cognitive behavioral therapy (CBT) has been found to be effective in treating social anxiety, or what is commonly referred to as shyness. Shy people often turn to drinking to facilitate social interaction. But a better course of action (as opposed to trying to hide the problem or "treat" it by drinking) would be to seek out a therapist who has expertise in helping individuals overcome their social anxiety. Without reaching out for help, it becomes a real challenge for anxious individuals and their partners to devise a lifestyle that avoids or copes with situations that trigger anxiety.

DEPRESSION

There's an old adage about people "drowning their sorrows" in alcohol. This attests to just how long people have turned to drinking to essentially help erase the depression that, like anxiety, may hang over them like a cloud. Just as people have long attempted to cope with anxiety by drinking, so have they resorted to alcohol in an attempt to escape depression. The irony is that alcohol is a depressant, so while temporary relief might be found through drinking, in the long run, alcohol will almost certainly worsen the depression.

Here again, a collaborative approach may be the best approach for couples, relying on sober love to help them embrace an identity as a sober couple. The depressed individual, much like the anxious person, may be reluctant to admit to suffering from depression—or even recognize the symptoms for what they are. Their partners, though, may have a more accurate perception of their emotional state. Admitting to depression can be difficult. Its causes can range from lifestyle issues such as a failed relationship, to physical issues such as poor health or disability, to more existential issues such as a lack of a sense of meaning.

Today, the recognized approach to dealing with depression is to combine medication with psychotherapy. Several psychotherapeutic approaches have been studied and found to be helpful in this regard (see the appendix). Either approach alone—medication or psychotherapy—is not likely as effective as the two in combination. Having the support of a loving partner, who understands the role that depression can play in leading to drinking and who supports dealing with it head-on, can be nothing short of lifesaving, as the example of Peter and Marie below shows.

CONFRONTING THE EMOTIONAL CONTEXT OF DRINKING

It isn't hard to understand why individuals who are burdened with anxiety or depression might turn to drinking as a source of comfort. Again, at the low-risk level, alcohol can have a comforting effect, and it's been used that way for centuries. When a person uses alcohol to deal with chronic anxiety or depression, however, their drinking can gradually progress along the substance use spectrum, from mild to severe, especially among those men and women who are constitutionally able to build a tolerance to alcohol or whose social networks strongly support their drinking.

Working through the emotional context of slips and slides begins, as with the other contexts, with some insight. Couples are wise to devote some time to taking stock of their lifestyles to determine whether depression or anxiety might be an issue for one of them. If that turns out to be the case in your relationship, the solution lies in facing the problem head-on, and then taking steps to effectively eliminate it.

PETER AND MARIE

Peter, 69, had retired from his job as an engineer two years earlier. For more than 40 years, he had been the main provider for his family and was a respected professional at work. His wife, Marie, had retired not long after Peter did. Since retiring, she watched her 3-year-old granddaughter part time. That required Marie to travel an hour and a half, so she often spent one night a week in her daughter's spare bedroom. She was also active in several church-related activities, such as clothing and food drives. Peter, however, had less going on. He described his new lifestyle this way: "I watch our two dogs,

sometimes read books, but mostly watch the news. That's about it."
It was evident as he described this lifestyle that Peter was currently
somewhat bored and depressed.

For most of their marriage, both Peter and Marie had been regular drinkers. While Peter favored gin and tonic, Marie preferred red
wine. They both could admit that their drinking had increased after
they retired, though not to the point where either of them recognized
it as a problem. But Peter was in fact already in the mild problem zone
on the spectrum, and moving quickly toward the moderate zone.
Whereas he'd once indulged in his gin and tonic largely on weekends,
he now had them almost daily while sitting home and doing nothing
much more than watching television. He was beginning to develop
a habit of "topping off" his drink with some gin while it was still
half full, and Marie was now having at least one if not more glasses
of Cabernet every day, starting before dinner. So far, the main consequence that they could have reasonably connected to their drinking was chronic fitful sleep that left them both feeling somewhat
lethargic, but they attributed that to aging rather than drinking.
Marie, however, had noted a slow but seemingly steady darkening
in her husband's personality. For example, he began criticizing Marie for almost any purchases she made, arguing that she was being
extravagant. She also felt that Peter sometimes picked arguments
with her for no apparent reason, or over some minor issue, like her
response to a television newscast.

Aside from having retired from an intellectually challenging job,
Peter had at one time had a few good male friends, including two he
played golf with weekly. Unfortunately, one of these friends had died,
and another had moved to a warmer climate. His contact with the
lone remaining friend had gradually fallen by the wayside, though
Peter had no good explanation for why.

Marie felt responsible for helping Peter climb out of the depression, lethargy, and irritability that he had fallen victim to. She decided to confront him, saying that it bothered her deeply to see the husband whom she knew to be so intelligent and productive slip into a state she described as "vegetative." Moreover, she said she was beginning to worry about Peter's physical and mental health if he did not do something to help himself. Most importantly, Marie raised the issue of drinking and questioned whether Peter's depression and lack of energy were connected to his several drinks a day, on top of his new restricted lifestyle.

The first step Peter took in response to Marie's observations was to reach out to his one remaining male friend and suggest they meet for lunch. The friend responded that he had missed their former regular contact and was happy to meet, hoping that they could rekindle the friendship. It was during that lunch that the friend asked Peter if he'd read any interesting history books lately. Peter had a long-standing avocation as a student of history, in particular American history. He'd always been a voracious reader, but recently he had let that gradually slip away too. It had become too difficult to keep focus while reading, especially after a few gin and tonics. Peter admitted that he'd pretty much let all of his interests go, and that making this contact with his friend was his first step toward breaking out of his isolation.

Then Peter's friend took a step further and mentioned that he and his wife had made a decision to stop drinking. They had come to realize that they had come to drink "quite a bit" since retiring, and that one consequence was that his wife had been diagnosed with high blood pressure. Her doctor connected her condition to drinking.

His friend's comment stuck with Peter. He mulled it over, then one night brought it up with Marie. To his surprise, she said that she had been thinking the same thing for a while, particularly the fact that she did not sleep as well or feel as energized as she once did. Recently she had begun to recognize a connection with her own increased drinking.

Following a second conversation a week later, Peter and Marie decided that they too would stop drinking, at least for the time being. They did not think that their decision would cause any significant problems for them in their limited social circle, which included some couples who drank quite a bit and others who drank very little.

To finish this story, part of Peter's solution to his depression (which he felt was linked to his increased drinking) was to join a number of online chat groups devoted to American history. In addition, he found that there was a museum nearby that focused on Civil War history, including memorabilia, dioramas depicting key battles, and artwork from the period. He signed up to be a docent at the museum once a month, and found his new job to be very satisfying.

MOVING FORWARD

If there is a lesson to be learned from this chapter, it's that slips and slides don't simply fall out of the sky. They are not random events, nor do they occur outside of any context. Couples seeking a sober identity can benefit from understanding the three contexts of slips and slides:

- Cognitive context: What were you thinking?
- Social context: Where were you and who were you with?
- Emotional context: What were you feeling?

Armed with this insight, the person who has slipped, along with his or her partner, can work collaboratively to anticipate and minimize such events moving forward. That all depends, however, on the recovering individual's and couple's willingness to embrace this view of slips and be prepared to act on it.

Before moving on to a discussion of yet another tool that sober couples have to help them achieve their goal—medication—it's important to keep slips and slides in perspective. First, making mistakes is hardly a new or unexpected phenomenon. Anyone who takes the time to check out any of the many supportive fellowships reviewed in this book will discover that one thing they have in common is the notion of "progress, not perfection." In other words, they all recognize the reality of being human. The best approach to dealing with a slip is to understand it and reach out for support in staying sober. It should not be simply swept under the rug, and it should never be cause for despair. In chapter 8, we made an inventory of the progress that you as a couple have made in achieving your goal. Do not let a slip negate your progress!

Chapter 15

MEDICATIONS FOR DRINKING

What You Need to Know

THE PRACTICE OF TRYING to help individuals who are addicted to one substance by substituting another less dangerous one, or by prescribing a medication to reduce cravings, has a substantial history. Today, this practice is known as medication-assisted treatment, or MAT. The US Food and Drug Administration (FDA) defines MAT as "the use of medications in combination with counseling and behavioral therapies, which is effective in the treatment of substance use disorders (SUD) and can help some people to sustain recovery."

The FDA regards MAT as part of a comprehensive treatment plan aimed at recovery (sobriety), one that also includes therapy. In other words, if MAT is to be part of a sobriety goal, it should not be used in isolation, but in combination with counseling aimed at making the kind of lifestyle changes we've discussed in this book. Recovery fellowships are an invaluable asset in that effort. If you recall, for several of the couples highlighted in this book, medication along with an abstinence-based fellowship and various lifestyle renovations and other changes worked in concert to help them become a sober couple.

MEDICATIONS FOR ALCOHOL USE DISORDER

Below we discuss some of the medications that are commonly prescribed to help individuals succeed in their pursuit of a sober lifestyle. Depending on where they fall on the drinking spectrum, along with their experience in being able to resist a drink, individuals and even couples may wish to discuss these options with their doctor.

NALTREXONE AND ACAMPROSATE

The most commonly prescribed medications to help individuals with alcohol use disorders stay sober are naltrexone and acamprosate. Naltrexone can be taken in two forms: as a tablet taken daily by mouth, or through a monthly injection under the brand name Vivitrol. Naltrexone and acamprosate (available under the brand name Campral) are also sometimes used in the treatment of opioid dependence. With respect to alcohol, naltrexone works by blocking the euphoric effects associated with intoxication, whereas acamprosate helps to reduce cravings. Research shows naltrexone and acamprosate are effective in helping individuals stay sober, but compliance rates for both medications tend to be low. In other words, many people who are prescribed naltrexone or acamprosate do not take it daily or consistently as prescribed, thereby limiting the drugs' effectiveness.

Clinicians frequently report that newly sober patients who are prescribed naltrexone or acamprosate take the medication as prescribed for a limited time, and then take it either inconsistently or not at all. Such compliance ("adherence" in medical terms) problems are not unique to these medications; rather, it is a common phenomenon associated with all sorts of medications prescribed for chronic conditions such as asthma and hypertension. Like these conditions, moderate to severe alcohol use is indeed a chronic condition. Just as a patient who is prescribed medication for hypertension may not meet with their prescriber often, so the individual who is prescribed naltrexone may not be followed closely. In both cases, over time, the patient may take the medication either inconsistently or not at all.

Planned Intoxication

Some individuals who are prescribed naltrexone (as well as disulfiram; see below) plan ahead of time to drink. For example, they may stop taking the medication on a Thursday in anticipation of going to a social event on Saturday and drinking. Under such circumstances, it would be inaccurate to argue in that case that the naltrexone "was not working." Instead, that is a case of the patient not "working the treatment."

An injectable, long-lasting form of naltrexone called Vivitrol was recently approved for use in the treatment of alcohol dependence. Like the oral form of naltrexone, it does not result in alcohol tolerance (the need for progressively more alcohol to produce the same effect). Like the oral form of naltrexone, the injectable form reduces the feelings of euphoria associated with intoxication. This longer-lasting option holds promise for people for whom compliance may be an issue. Because it is an injectable medication, the patient must visit a clinic or prescriber monthly in order to get their medication. This in itself may help to increase medication compliance—and, by implication, this medication's effectiveness.

DISULFIRAM (ANTABUSE)

Disulfiram—also known as Antabuse—is an oral medication that is taken daily. If a person has a drink after taking disulfiram, they will experience extreme discomfort, including nausea, vomiting, headache, and general weakness. After taking this medication, drinking becomes very uncomfortable. Still, some people may choose to take this medication simply because they are motivated to stop drinking. That is especially true for those who fall at the extreme end of the drinking spectrum, who most likely have experienced many unsuccessful attempts to stop drinking and are now determined to quit once and for all. Disulfiram is sometimes prescribed along with naltrexone in an effort to maximize a person's resistance to drinking.

GABAPENTIN

Gabapentin was initially developed and used to treat neurological disorders such as nerve pain and peripheral neuropathy, which can be caused by spinal stenosis or degenerative disk disease. It has also been found to be helpful in treating mild to moderate alcohol use disorder. It has a calming effect, can help improve sleep, and reduces cravings. But gabapentin is not recommended as a first-line treatment option for those with a severe drinking problem. Like the other drugs reviewed here, gabapentin is sometimes prescribed in combination with another drug.

SUMMING UP

It is of course up to the individual to decide whether adding a medication to their pursuit of a sober lifestyle is right for them. For couples who want to achieve sobriety together, medication may be an important topic for discussion. Some of the couples in this book considered medication when one partner found themselves much further along on the drinking spectrum than the other. Repeated failures at trying to stop (or "control") drinking are discouraging to say the least. In that case, sober love may come into play: a decision to take medication because an individual cares enough not only about themselves, but also about their relationship.

Chapter 16

BEYOND A DRINKING CULTURE

AS IS EVIDENT THROUGHOUT this book, one of the reasons it is so hard to stop drinking is because of the *drinking culture* we live in. Through advertising, product placement, and even news stories about the supposed "benefits" of alcohol, the liquor industry promotes drinking as normal, expected behavior. In fact, those who choose to abstain are often considered to be the abnormal ones.

The pressure our culture puts on us to drink starts at an early age. According to the National Center for Drug Abuse Statistics, drug use by eighth graders increased by 61% between 2016 and 2020. As for drinking, 1.19 *million* 12- to 17-year-olds and a whopping 11.72 *million* 18- to 25-year-olds reported binge drinking in the last *month*. (The Centers for Disease Control and Prevention defines binge drinking as having five or more drinks on one occasion.) You read it correctly: *millions* of young people have engaged in dangerous binge drinking in the past *month* alone. Taken together, the data we have about alcohol strongly support the idea that "America has a drinking problem," as was argued in *The Atlantic* article cited at the beginning of this book. Indeed, America today is awash in drinking.

THE STORY DOESN'T END HERE

Unfortunately, alcohol is not the only problem facing Americans today. The focus of this book has been on drinking and how couples who care enough about their relationship can work toward being sober together. But we would be remiss if we did not expand the scope of the discussion to some other substances that can have a negative effect on people's lives.

CANNABIS

Sticking with youths for the time being, studies have found that as many as 7% of twelfth graders report smoking pot *daily*, and more than 30% have smoked it within the past year. Among adults, daily cannabis use has risen steadily from 2002 to 2014, with roughly 15% of adults stating they were regular (weekly or daily) users. Cannabis is currently legally available, either medicinally or recreationally, in more than 40 US states or districts.

The US cannabis industry is projected to reach $72 billion annually by 2030. The industry promotes cannabis use in much the same way the alcohol industry does drinking, as normal, harmless, and even helpful for relieving pain and producing a calming effect. But there is scarce mention in their promotions (just like liquor ads) of the potential for negative effects or addiction. That has been true for many substances that were once touted as "harmless and helpful," including cocaine and prescription opioids, both of which turned out to have decidedly dark sides.

There are no medical standards for dosage or even indicated conditions for cannabis, nor is there research on the more than 100 other cannabinoids (besides THC) that the marijuana plant contains. Meanwhile, warning signs are emerging. A study published in *JAMA*

Pediatrics, for example, reported that the children of women who consumed cannabis during pregnancy are at greater risk for mental health and substance use disorders in their teenage years. As for adults, accumulating research supports the idea that cannabis follows the same pathway to addiction as other drugs, including tolerance, negative neurological consequences, impaired functioning, and severe withdrawal.

BENZODIAZEPINES

Benzodiazepines, or "benzos," as they are commonly called, have long been prescribed to treat anxiety. Like all other mood-altering substances, they were initially promoted by their manufacturers as "harmless and helpful," with little to no mention of misuse or the possibility of addiction. The truth is that many individuals come to rely on benzos on a regular basis, to the tune of nearly 31 million men and women. Many obtain them by prescription, though an increasing number access benzos in other ways. Some studies have found a link between the use of cannabis or alcohol and an increased use of benzos. Moreover, it appears that many individuals consider benzo use as harmless despite their reliance on it. Oftentimes benzos are used as a sleep aid. But it could be that some users have disrupted sleep because of their drinking.

OPIOIDS

The United States is currently experiencing a major crisis involving the misuse of prescription and nonprescription opioids, including heroin, oxycontin, and fentanyl. Overdoses and deaths associated with this supposedly "helpful and harmless" substance increased by 30% from 2019 to 2020, and in 2020 there were more than 90,000 reported overdose deaths. Opioids, much like crack cocaine, often quickly lead users down a "slippery slope" along the substance use spectrum, from low-risk or "experimental" use to full-blown addiction. Unfortunately, many of those addicted to opioids believe that they can drink safely, ignoring the fact that alcohol has long been known to disinhibit behavior ranging from violence to sex to drug use.

THE CHALLENGES AND REWARDS OF CHOOSING TO BE A SOBER COUPLE

I include this discussion of substances besides alcohol to emphasize just how challenging it can be for a couple to embrace an identity as a sober couple amid a culture full of substance use. As the title of another chapter suggests, the strategies for pursuing sober love are much like "coloring outside the lines." It is truly going against the grain to live a sober lifestyle.

Being a sober couple involves much more than simply not drinking. It means immersing yourselves in a new lifestyle that is richer and more rewarding than the reduced and hollowed-out drinking lifestyle where shared pleasures become a rarity and the common ground that connects a couple shrinks. Becoming a sober couple means substituting thoughts about (and cravings for) a drink—which in essence is a distraction—with living in and enjoying the here and now.

The couples' stories in this book all attest to the awakening associated with a new lifestyle that comes through sober love. My hope is that you and your partner will discover in these stories valuable information that can help you in planning for a new identity as a sober couple.

ACKNOWLEDGMENTS

If it takes a village to raise a child, then it takes a team to produce a book. I'd like to acknowledge that team:

Linda Konner, my long-standing agent, for her steadfast faith in me through thick and thin (in other words, rejection and acceptance).

Suzanne Staszak-Silva, senior editor at Johns Hopkins University Press, for shepherding *Sober Love* from proposal to acceptance.

Ashleigh McKown, copy editor extraordinaire, for her thorough and skillful editing as well as her thoughtful questions.

Kyle Kretzer, senior production editor, for organizing and supervising a production process that is much more complex than it might seem.

Kathy Patterson, for a most user-friendly index.

Diem Bloom, director of publishing operations, for putting the whole production effort together.

Marvin Seppala, MD, for taking the time to thoroughly read the manuscript and write his generous foreword.

Appendix

SOURCES AND FURTHER READING

This appendix contains references and links to the resources that are described or cited in the book, for readers who wish to peruse this material in greater depth. They are organized by chapter, beginning with the introduction. You can access these sources by searching the agencies' websites or via the provided links.

INTRODUCTION. WHY THIS BOOK, AND WHY NOW?

The following sources provide data on alcohol-related deaths:

Centers for Disease Control and Prevention. "Deaths from Excessive Alcohol Use in the United States." Last reviewed July 6, 2022. https://www.cdc.gov/alcohol/features/excessive-alcohol -deaths.html#print.

Julian, Kate. "America Has a Drinking Problem." *The Atlantic* (July/August 2021): https://www.theatlantic.com/magazine /archive/2021/07/america-drinking-alone-problem/619017/.

National Institute on Alcohol Abuse and Alcoholism. *Trends in Alcohol-Related Morbidity among Community Hospital Discharges, United States, 2000–2015*. Surveillance Report 112. Bethesda, MD: NIAAA, 2018.

On defining a "standard drink," see:

National Institute on Alcohol Abuse and Alcoholism. "Rethinking Drinking: Alcohol and Your Health." Accessed September 19, 2023. https://www.rethinkingdrinking.niaaa.nih.gov/.

One comprehensive review calls into question the popular notion that so-called moderate drinking has beneficial effects on health:

Zhao, Jinhui, Tim Stockwell, Tim Naimi, Sam Churchill, James Clay, and Adam Sherk. "A Systematic Review and Meta-Analyses." *JAMA Network Open* 6, no. 3 (2023): https://jamanetwork.com/journals/jamanetworkopen/fullarticle/2802963.

For more information on women with alcohol use disorders and their partners, see:

McCrady, Barbara S., Elizabeth E. Epstein, Sharon Cook, Noelle Jensen, and Thomas Hildebrant. "A Randomized Trial of Individual and Couple Behavioral Alcohol Treatment for Women." *Journal of Consulting and Clinical Psychology* 77, no. 2 (2009): 243–56. https://doi.org/10.1037/a0014686.

O'Farrell, Timothy J., and W. Fals-Stewart. "Behavioral Couples Therapy for Alcoholism and Drug Abuse." *Journal of Substance Abuse Treatment* 18, no. 1 (2000): 51–54. https://doi.org/10.1016/s0740-5472(99)00026-4.

CHAPTER 1. IT'S ABOUT LOVE

Nowinski, Joseph. "What Is Your 'Relationship' with Alcohol?" *Psychology Today*, May 19, 2012. https://www.psychologytoday.com/us/blog/the-almost-effect/201205/what-is-your-relationship-alcohol.

CHAPTER 2. WHY WE DRINK

For data relative to advertising and youthful drinking, see:

Snyder, Leslie B., Frances Fleming Milici, Michael Slater, Helen Sun, and Yuliya Strizhakova. "Effects of Alcohol Advertising Exposure on Drinking Among Youth." *Archives of Pediatrics and Adolescent Medicine* 160, no. 1 (2006):18–24. https://doi .org/10.1001/archpedi.160.1.18.

On advertising expenditures by the alcohol industry, see:

Carruthers, Nicola. "Alcohol Ad Spend to Hit $6bn by 2023." *Spirits Business*, May 24, 2021. https://www.thespiritsbusiness .com/2021/05/alcohol-ad-spend-to-hit-6bn-by-2023/.
Knapp, Carolyn. *Drinking: A Love Story.* New York: Dial Press, 1997.

For information on the genetics of alcoholism among first- and second-degree relatives, see:

Dawson, D. A., T. C. Harford, and B. F. Grant. "Family History as a Predictor of Alcohol Dependence." *Alcoholism: Clinical and Experimental Research* 16, no. 3 (1992): 572–75. https://pubmed .ncbi.nlm.nih.gov/1626658/.

For information on the genetics of alcoholism among identical twins, see:

Heath, Andrew C. "Genetic Influences on Alcoholism Risk." *Alcohol Health and Research World* 19, no. 3. (1995): 166–71. https://www.ncbi.nlm.nih.gov/pmc/articles/PMC6875767/.

CHAPTER 4. WHAT IT TAKES

The following sources include research on controlled drinking:

Bujarski, Spencer, Stephanie S. O'Malley, Katy Lunny, and Lara A. Ray. "The Effects of Drinking Goal on Treatment Outcome for Alcoholism." *Journal of Consulting and Clinical Psychology* 81, no. 1 (2013): 13–22.

Humphreys, Keith. "Alcohol and Drug Abuse: A Research-Based Analysis of the Moderation Management Controversy." *Psychiatric Services* 54, no. 5 (2003): 621–22. https://doi.org/10 .1176/appi.ps.54.5.621.

Miller, W. R., A. L. Leckman, H. D. Delaney, and M. Tinkcom. "Long-Term Follow-Up of Behavioral Self-Control Training." *Journal of Studies on Alcohol* 53, no. 3 (1992): 249–61.

For information on drinking patterns in older adults, see:

Barnes, A. J., A. A. Moore, H. Xu, A. Ang, L. Tallen, M. Mirkin, and S. L. Ettner. "Prevalence and Correlates of At-Risk Drinking among Older Adults: The Project SHARE Study." *Journal of General Internal Medicine* 25 (2010): 840–46. https://link .springer.com/article/10.1007/s11606-010-1341-x.

Han, B. H., A. A. Moore, R. Ferris, and J. J. Palamar. "Binge Drinking among Older Adults in the United States, 2015 to 2017." *Journal of the American Geriatric Society* 67, no. 10 (2019): 2139–44. https://www.ncbi.nlm.nih.gov/pmc/articles /PMC6800799/.

For research on psychological hardiness, see:

Judkins, Jason L., and Brian A. Moore. "Psychological Hardiness." *Psychology in the Real Word*, May 29, 2022. https://www

.researchgate.net/publication/339882546_Psychological
   _Hardiness.

Kobasa, Suzanne C. "Stressful Life Events, Personality, and Health:
   An Inquiry into Hardiness." *Journal of Personality and Social
   Psychology* 37, no. 1 (1979): 1–11. https://doi.org/10.1037/0022
   -3514.37.1.1.

Kobasa, Suzanne C., Salvatore R. Maddi, and Stephen Kahn.
   "Hardiness and Health: A Prospective Study." *Journal of
   Personality and Social Psychology* 42, no. 1 (1982): 168–77.
   https://doi.org/10.1037/0022-3514.42.1.168.

For the results of Alcoholics Anonymous membership surveys, see:

Alcoholics Anonymous. "Estimated Worldwide AA Individual and
   Group Membership." Accessed September 20, 2023. https://
   www.aa.org/sites/default/files/literature/smf-132_Estimated
   _Membership_EN_1221.pdf.

Mehdikhani, M. "AA Membership Survey 2020." Alcoholics
   Anonymous, accessed September 20, 2023. https://www
   .alcoholics-anonymous.org.uk/download/1/documents
   /AA%20Membership%20Survey%202020.pdf.

The following sources provide information on the effectiveness of Alcoholics Anonymous:

Kelly, John F., Keith Humphreys, and Marica Ferri. "Alcoholics
   Anonymous and Other 12-Step Programs for Alcohol Use
   Disorder." *Cochrane Database of Systematic Reviews* 3 (2020):
   CD012880. https://www.cochranelibrary.com/cdsr/doi/10
   .1002/14651858.CD012880.pub2/full.

McCarthy, Moira. "Alcoholics Anonymous Is Most Effective
   Treatment for Addiction, Researchers Say." Healthline,

March 11, 2020. https://www.healthline.com/health-news
/alcoholics-anonymous-is-still-the-most-effective-way-to-deal
-with-alcohol-addiction.

Nowinski, J. *The Twelve Step Facilitation Handbook: A Therapeutic
Approach to Treatment and Recovery*, 2nd ed. Center City, MN:
Hazelden, 2018.

CHAPTER 5. A NEW IDENTITY

Erikson, Erik. *Identity: Youth and Crisis*. New York: W. W. Norton,
1968.

On Dr. Marsha Linehan's epiphany, see:

Carey, Benedict. "Expert on Mental Illness Reveals Her Own
Fight." *New York Times*, June 23, 2011. http://www.nytimes.com
/2011/06/23/health/23lives.html?pagewanted=all&_r=0.

On Malcolm X and epiphany, see:

Haley, Alex. *The Autobiography of Malcolm X*. New York: Ballan-
tine Books, 1992.

Check out the following for information on supportive fellowships:

Alcoholics Anonymous (www.aa.org)
Alcoholics Anonymous. *Alcoholics Anonymous*, 4th ed. New York:
Alcoholics Anonymous World Services, 2001.
Recovering Couples Anonymous (https://recovering-couples.org)
Secular AA (www.aasecular.org)
Joe C. *Beyond Belief: Agnostic Musings for 12 Step Life*. Picton, ON:
Rebellion Dogs, 2013.
SMART Recovery (http://smartrecovery.org)

Hardin, Rosemary. *SMART Recovery Handbook*, 3rd ed. Mentor,
   OH: Adashn Incorporated, 2013.
The Red Road to Recovery (www.theredroad.org)
White Bison. *The Red Road to Wellbriety: In the Native American
   Way.* Colorado Springs: Coyhis Publishing, 2015.
Women for Sobriety (https://womenforsobriety.org)
Fitzpatrick, Jean. *Women for Sobriety: The Program Booklet.*
   Quakertown, PA: Women for Sobriety, 2017.

CHAPTER 7. A RECIPE FOR SUCCESS

Piper, W. *The Little Engine That Could.* New York: Golden Books
   Reprint, 2021.

On the role of self-efficacy in promoting a sober lifestyle, see:

Buckingham, S. A., D. Frings, and I. P. Albery. "Group Membership
   and Social Identity in Addiction Recovery." *Psychology of
   Addictive Behaviors* 27, no. 4 (2013): 1132–40.
Maddux, James E. "Self-Efficacy: The Power of Believing You
   Can." In *The Handbook of Positive Psychology*, 227–87. Oxford:
   Oxford University Press, 2012. https://www.researchgate
   .net/publication/285193896_Self-Efficacy_The_Power_of
   _Believing_You_Can.

On the role of social support in promoting a sober lifestyle, see:

Kelly, John F., Keith Humphreys, and Marica Ferri. "Alcoholics
   Anonymous and Other 12-Step Programs for Alcohol Use
   Disorder." *Cochrane Database of Systematic Reviews* 3 (2020):
   CD012880. https://www.cochranelibrary.com/cdsr/doi/10
   .1002/14651858.CD012880.pub2/full.

McCarthy, Moira. "Alcoholics Anonymous Is Most Effective Treatment for Addiction, Researchers Say." Healthline, March 11, 2020. https://www.healthline.com/health-news /alcoholics-anonymous-is-still-the-most-effective-way-to-deal -with-alcohol-addiction.

CHAPTER 10. REKINDLING INTIMACY

Masters, W., and V. Johnson. *Human Sexual Inadequacy.* Bronx, NY: Ishi Press, 2010. (Previously published by Little, Brown in 1970).

Stopes, Marie. *Married Love.* Oxford: Oxford University Press, 2004. (First published in 1918.)

CHAPTER 11. SPIRITUALITY AND SOBER LOVE

Research on spirituality and sobriety can be found in the following sources:

Carroll, S. "Spirituality and Purpose in Life in Alcoholism Recovery." *Journal of Studies on Alcoholism* 54 (1993): 297–301.

Galanter, M. "Research on Spirituality and Alcoholics Anonymous." *Alcoholism: Clinical and Experimental Research* 23, no. 4 (1999): 716–19.

Kelly, J. F., R. L. Stout, M. Magill, J. S. Tonigan, and M. E. Pagano. "Spirituality in Recovery: A Lagged Mediational Analysis of Alcoholics Anonymous' Principal Theoretical Mechanism of Behavior Change." *Alcoholism: Clinical and Experimental Research* 35, no. 3 (2011): 454–63.

Mathew, R. J., J. Georgi, W. H. Wilson, and V. G. Mathew. "A Retrospective Study of the Concept of Spirituality as Understood by Recovering Alcoholics." *Journal of Substance Abuse Treatment* 13, no. 1 (1995): 67–73.

CHAPTER 12. COLORING OUTSIDE THE LINES

For a review of the research on self-efficacy, see:

Pajares, Frank. "Current Directions in Self-Efficacy Research." Dynaread. Accessed September 20, 2023. https://www .dynaread.com/current-directions-in-self-efficacy-research.

CHAPTER 14. SLIPPING AND SLIDING

For information on cognitive behavioral therapy for anxiety, see:

Bunmi O., J. Olatunji, Brett Cisler, and J. Deacon. "Efficacy of Cognitive Behavioral Therapy for Anxiety Disorders: A Review of Meta-Analytic Findings." *Psychiatric Clinics of North America* 33, no. 3 (2010): 557–77.

For information on psychotherapy for depression, see:

Cuijpers, P., A. van Straten, G. Andersson, and P. van Oppen. "Psychotherapy for Depression in Adults: A Meta-Analysis of Comparative Outcome Studies." *Journal of Consulting and Clinical Psychology* 76, no. 6 (2008): 909–22.

CHAPTER 15. MEDICATIONS FOR DRINKING

The following resources have information on the efficacy of medication for alcohol abuse:

Bouza, Carmen, Magro Angeles, Ana Muñoz, and José María Amate. "Efficacy and Safety of Naltrexone and Acamprosate in

the Treatment of Alcohol Dependence: A Systematic Review."
Addiction 99 (2004): 811–28.

Dermody, Sarah S., Jeffery D. Wardell, Susan A. Stoner, and
Christian S. Hendershot. "Predictors of Daily Adherence to
Naltrexone for Alcohol Use Disorder Treatment during a
Mobile Health Intervention." *Annals of Behavioral Medicine* 52,
no. 9 (2018): 787–97. https://www.ncbi.nlm.nih.gov/pmc
/articles/PMC6105286/.

Palpacuer, C., R. Duprez, A. Huneau, C. Locher, R. Boussageon,
B. Laviolle, and F. Naudet. "Pharmacologically Controlled
Drinking in the Treatment of Alcohol Dependence or Alcohol
Use Disorders: A Systematic Review with Direct and Network
Meta-Analyses on Nalmefene, Naltrexone, Acamprosate,
Baclofen and Topiramate." *Addiction* 113, no. 2 (2018): 220–37.
https://pubmed.ncbi.nlm.nih.gov/28940866/.

Perez-Macia, Virginia, Mireia Martinez-Cotes, Jesus Mesones,
Manuel Segura-Trepichio, and Lorena Garcia-Fernandez.
"Monitoring and Improving Naltrexone Adherence in Patients
with Substance Use Disorder." *Patient Preference and Adherence* 15 (2021): 999–1015. https://www.ncbi.nlm.nih.gov/pmc
/articles/PMC8140930/.

Substance Abuse and Mental Health Services Administration.
"What Is Naltrexone?" Last updated September 18, 2023.
https://www.samhsa.gov/medication-assisted-treatment
/medications-counseling-related-conditions/naltrexone.

Swift, Robert, David W. Oslin, Mark Alexander, and Robert
Forman. "Adherence Monitoring in Naltrexone Pharmaco-
therapy Trials: A Systematic Review." *Journal of Studies on
Alcohol and Drugs* 72, no. 6 (2011): 1012–18. https://www.jsad
.com/doi/abs/10.15288/jsad.2011.72.1012.

CHAPTER 16. BEYOND A
DRINKING CULTURE

See the following sources for data on opioid-related deaths:

Centers for Disease Control and Prevention. "Understanding the Opioid Overdose Epidemic." Last reviewed August 8, 2023. https://www.cdc.gov/opioids/basics/epidemic.html.

National Center for Health Statistics. "Drug Overdose Deaths in the U.S. Top 100,000 Annually." Press release, November 17, 2021. https://www.cdc.gov/nchs/pressroom/nchs_press _releases/2021/20211117.htm.

Planalp, C., R. Hest, and M. Lahr. *The Opioid Epidemic: National Trends in Opioid-Related Overdose Deaths from 2000 to 2017*. Princeton, NJ: Robert Wood Johnson Foundation, June 2019. http://resource.nlm.nih.gov/101753751.

US Department of Health and Human Services. "Opioid Facts and Statistics." Last reviewed December 16, 2022. https://www .hhs.gov/opioids/statistics/index.html.

For information on cannabis dependence, see:

Budney, A. J., R. Roffman, R. S. Stephens, and D. Walker. "Marijuana Dependence and Its Treatment." *Addiction Science and Clinical Practice* 4, no. 1 (2007): 4–16. https://www.ncbi.nlm .nih.gov/pmc/articles/PMC2797098/.

Zehra, A., J. Burns, C. K. Liu, P. Manza, C. E. Wiers, M. D. Volkow, and G.-J. Wang. "Cannabis Addiction and the Brain: A Review." *Journal of Neuroimmune Pharmacology* 13 (2018): 438–52. https://link.springer.com/article/10.1007/S11481 -018-9782-9.

For information on benzodiazepine dependence, see:

American Addiction Centers. "Benzodiazepine Addiction: Symptoms and Signs of Dependence." Last updated September 15, 2022. https://americanaddictioncenters.org/benzodiazepine /symptoms-and-signs.

INDEX

abstinence, 58, 138-39; as "abnormal" behavior, 17-18, 31, 37, 112-13, 128, 135, 136, 178; "controlled" drinking vs., 42-43, 58, 83, 90, 133, 157-58; cultural attitudes toward, 18; percentage of days abstinent (PDA), 122-24, 139, 140. *See also* recovery fellowships; sobriety / sober love

acamprosate (Campral), 175-76, 193-94

accidental injuries, alcohol use-related, 8, 12, 63

accommodation of drinking, 91-101, 120; case studies, 87-100, 103-13, 145-54

adolescents and young adults: alcohol advertising targeted to, 16, 17, 187; alcohol consumption levels, 16, 17, 178; with alcoholic parents, 68-69; binge drinking, 178; cannabis (marijuana) use, 179; onset age of alcohol use, 26, 32, 149, 178; social networks, 49-50; substance abuse disorders, 179-80

advertising: of alcoholic beverages, 16-17, 18, 22, 178, 187; of cannabis (marijuana), 179

Al-Anon, online resources, 72-73

alcohol blood level, 159

alcohol counselors, 163

alcohol dependence, 110

alcoholic beverages: advertising of, 16-17, 18, 22, 179, 187; alcohol content of "standard drinks," 2; availability in the home, 8, 9, 10, 32; drinks per drinking day (DDD), 122-24; nonalcoholic beverages as substitutes for, 99, 109, 114; purchase of, 10; removal from the home, 109, 114, 152; switching of brands or types, 54, 93, 94

Alcoholics Anonymous (AA), 23, 56, 58-59, 109-10, 128, 138, 152, 156, 158, 190; 12 Steps, 54-55, 56, 63-64; combined with counseling/therapy, 47-48, 152, 159-60; effectiveness, 138, 189-90; membership criterion,

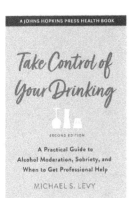

"A straightforward, practical approach to understanding and managing alcohol abuse and addiction from a nationally recognized leader in addiction medicine. A must-read for anyone struggling with alcohol abuse."

—Gary Gastman,
Executive Director, Link House

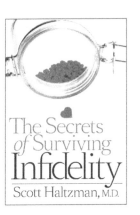

"This isn't *just* a supremely helpful book on understanding—and recovering from—infidelity. It's a great book on marriage. This is the book you are looking for right now."

—Scott Stanley, PhD,
author of *The Power of Commitment*

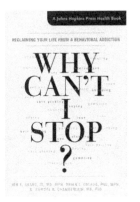

A life-changing book for anyone caught in the whirlpool of a behavioral addiction.

JOHNS HOPKINS UNIVERSITY PRESS

PRESS.JHU.EDU